# SEX & GERMS: THE POLITICS OF AIDS

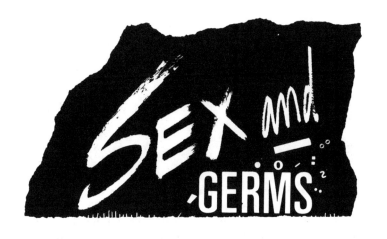

# THE POLITICS OF AIDS

Cindy Patton

**SOUTH END PRESS**　　　　　　**BOSTON**

First edition
Editing, typesetting, layout by South End Press, USA
Manufactured in the USA
Cover design by Tom Huth

Library of Congress Cataloguing in Publication Data

Patton, Cindy, 1955-
    Sex & Germs

    Bibliography: p. 175
    Includes index.
    1. AIDS (Disease)—Political aspects—United States.
2. AIDS (Disease)—Social aspects—United States.
3. Homosexuals—United States—Political activity.
I. Title. II. Titles: Sex and germs.
RA644.A25P38 1985          362.1'969792'00973          85-26240
ISBN 0-89608-260-1
ISBN 0-89608-259-8 (pbk.)
10 9 8 7 6 5 4 3 2

SOUTH END PRESS          116 St Botolph St          Boston MA 02115

## Dedication

*For the people with AIDS who have guided me through these past few years: Hoagy, Rita, Kevin, Michael, Terry, and Mark, with love.*

# Acknowledgments

I was afraid that writing this book might take me too far from the gritty, sad AIDS organizing work. But many events—some described in the Epilogue—convinced me that this book might provide a beginning in the necessary process of understanding what AIDS means for the many kinds of people affected, and might create a vision of what the post-AIDS lesbian and gay consciousness might be like.

Many people encouraged me when I was uncertain, and pulled me back to earth when I became too delighted with abstract theories. I take ultimate responsibility for the project, however, because the book reflects what I experienced working on and thinking about AIDS from the summer of 1981 until the summer of 1985, when I shipped the manuscript off to the printer.

My parents may have preferred that I write a different book, one that required fewer explanations if shown to friends. I hope they will see in these pages the love of community, respect for individuals, and belief in the essential goodness of peoples, which they taught me.

Carol Baker, my editor at South End Press, deserves much gratitude. Not only did she improve my prose, she showed me that writers and editors can share the writing process. I hope her faith in me is warranted.

My good friend Chris Guilfoy's excellent AIDS coverage in the *Gay Community News* was an invaluable resource. David Peterson's extensive files on the religious right were also extremely helpful. Bob Andrews and I spent three months in 1982-1983 writing an article about the impact of AIDS on the lesbian and gay community, a vision expanded in this book. Bob's friendship through the years and especially our work together on the AIDS Action Committee proved to me that lesbians and gay men can work together.

Tom Huth designed the cover of this book. His perfectionism kept me going through many drafts of the book. Our regular trips to the gym kept me sane.

Michael Bronski provided tea, distraction, access to his files, and most importantly, hours of frank discussion about sex.

Peg Byron gave me a great deal of information and moral support. She convinced me of the significance of AIDS when I was still a skeptic.

This book came together on an unusually rapid schedule, especially given the constantly changing medical and political implications. Joe Interrante and Janice Irvine served as readers virtually as the book went to press.

Finally, I want to thank my lover, Amy Hoffman. Her editorial assistance over the years, support of my work, and her own fiction and essays have given me a mark of excellence to strive toward, and gentle nurturance when I failed.

# Contents

# SECTION ONE
# Learning About AIDS

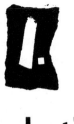

# Introduction

Many books have and will be written about AIDS; this is just one approach. It grew out of my experience as an AIDS activist and my concern for sexual freedom. I decided to write this book on AIDS and sexual politics because I had trouble convincing friends to approach AIDS organizing as a lesbian and gay liberation issue, and to get involved in the work. There was a variety of excuses—burnout from other political projects; a feeling that AIDS was affecting those *other* gay men, the non-political ones who had taken advantage of the gains of gay liberation without ever putting in any of the work; a sense of despair and isolation; an insularity that bred an attitude that there was no longer an identifiable gay movement. I had trouble reorienting my own worldview to bring gay liberation and AIDS organizing into focus within a single frame, so how could I convey this transformation of perspective to others? AIDS was not the anticipated "next step" in the march toward gay liberation, and yet the strength of the contemporary lesbian and gay movement would be judged by its response to AIDS.

The reluctance of many of my politically sophisticated friends to become actively involved in AIDS organizing signalled some threat buried deep in the issues and feelings which the appearance of AIDS had tapped. I began to see AIDS not just as another event in the lesbian and gay community, but as an important watershed in ideology and in the evolution of social and political power for lesbians and gay men in contemporary American society.

If we did not see the implications of AIDS for the future of lesbian and gay organizing, then the right wing certainly did. Clem Muller and

Paul Cameron, two doctors from the anti-gay Dallas Doctors Against
AIDS, said, "Such a severe public health concern must cause the citi-
zenry of this country to do everything in their power to smash the
homosexual movement in this country to make sure these kinds of acts
are criminalized."[1]

AIDS cannot be viewed outside the quest for sexual liberation.
Nowhere is the relationship between the rhetoric of liberation and the
everyday practice of sex more connected and more painful than when
formulating individual and community responses to AIDS. Questions
of whether, with whom, and how to have sex have loomed larger for gay
men in the four years that AIDS has been a medical and political reality.
But the matrix of analyses available for understanding the terror of
living under siege has proved incomplete, cumbersome, and sometimes
plain reactionary. How does anyone remain sex-positive when the
newspapers and passersby see homosexuals = AIDS = death?

A re-examination of the fear of germs and of the erotic fleshes out
the broader discussion of the meaning and role of AIDS to sexual
oppression and liberation. Individual responses to cultural notions of
sex and germs are related to the history of medicine, and to popular
ideas about what constitutes sickness and health. We need a new way of
understanding how germs—things we fear will invade our bodies from
the outside—and the erotic—the power that threatens to take over our
bodies from within—are politicized to exert social control over the
expression of our deepest fears and joys. The march of history which we
see in social and political events is interpenetrated by the physicality of
everyday life, yet our sense of physicality is much less articulated than
our understanding of the course of history. These two kinds of knowing
evolve by different rules: one moves in linear time, while the other—the
physical—is synchronous, making constant reference to the essential
aspects of human existence. AIDS activists are forced to understand the
interrelationship between sex and germs historically and intrapsychi-
cally if they are to evolve relevant strategies that will cope with the
immediate challenge of AIDS without sacrificing the broader cultural
and political aims which provide the framework for moving out of
individual despair to community strength and hope.

In both a profound and a practical sense, AIDS will not go away.
New and dramatic medical events like AIDS take decades or longer to
run their historical course to prevention and cure. The cultural lessons
and political realignments that result from AIDS organizing and from
the emotional impact of coping with an attack of such magnitude will
forever shade the picture of gay liberation history—as did the trial of
Oscar Wilde, the Stonewall riots, the banning of Radclyffe Hall's work,

the murder of Harvey Milk, or the emergence of "women's" music. But AIDS will be unique in its scope, degree, and possibilities for uniting or dividing elements of the lesbian and gay community—and in the necessity for negotiating with the very medical and governmental structures that have for so long oppressed lesbians and gay men.

## Learning about AIDS: the first step

My introduction to AIDS came while I was working as the features editor of Boston's *Gay Community News*. In July of 1981, I received a copy of the *Morbidity and Mortality Weekly Report*. The anonymous note bore only a red arrow, pointing to a report about six gay men in Los Angeles who had died of a rare pneumonia, *pneumocistis carinii* (PCP). My political and journalistic curiosities were piqued, so I called our local gay clinic, the public health department, and a doctor friend, none of whom had heard of this report. I wrote up a short news note, submitted it to the news editor, and put a red flag in my mental file for more information on this bizarre topic. At that time, my primary reaction was "how weird." I don't recall having felt any personal connection to those six dead gay men on the other coast. I did not know for over a year that while I pondered this abstraction, a close friend was becoming increasingly sick, and would ultimately be diagnosed with and die of AIDS. This experience of discovering information and then confronting its real life manifestation would be repeated for me at ever shortening intervals, and come increasingly closer to home. It seemed that every time I finished another article, or refined a new point of analysis, I would learn that another friend or political colleague had moved one step closer to a positive diagnosis, or one hospital episode closer to death.

The straight press began its assault soon after I discovered this first *MMWR* report. First "gay pneumonia," then "gay cancer"—when *Kaposi's sarcoma* (KS) was discovered in gay men in San Francisco and New York. Finally, "gay plague," when the list of attendant infections grew too numerous to include in a headline. I continued to file this information. I was not a gay man, and Boston is not New York, and I had yet to realize that *I* was under attack.

The reports in the mainstream press did not let up, although their frequency seemed to run in peaks and valleys precisely opposite to the real occurrence of events in the medical or gay male communities. AIDS impressionism caused editors and writers to include a story about AIDS as some curious insight struck them; only in 1984 did newspaper reports begin to bear any resemblance to what was actually happening. But if journalistic timing was now a little better, the facts were still transformed into wild notions bearing a closer resemblance to stereotypes about the affected groups than to scientific fact.

The mainstream press reports sounded as if AIDS were something you got for being gay. Mangled science reports laid the groundwork for twin misconceptions about the origin of AIDS that continue to be widely believed in both the lesbian/gay and straight populations (and maintained in anesthetized forms by some medical researchers). In one myth, AIDS is a disease of overindulgence. In the second, gay sexual activity is a sort of Russian roulette: perverse promiscuity is eventually bound to bring you in contact with a deadly germ.

Both of these ideas are problematic for a lesbian and gay community that is busy trying to gain acceptance, either from other progressives or from the mainstream liberals. At a time in lesbian and gay movement history when the trend is toward hiding or disguising *sex* under the rubric of "lifestyle," a "gay disease" that is somehow linked with sex is an embarrassment and a political liability. And lurking deep in the heart of even the most positive and progressive lesbians and gay men was the fear: maybe they are right, homosexuality is death.

## Media science

The media's popularized interpretations of medical research were all the more oppressive because they fit into the pre-existing fabric of prejudice about lesbians and gay men.[2]

Not surprisingly, the overload theories were the first posed, a reflection of the media success of the fast-lane, gay clone image in clothing and cigarette ads in lifestyle magazines.[3] The "clone revolution" consolidated the stereotype that gay men are superficial, concerned with beauty, live high for today, and disregard tomorrow.[4] These theories posited that gay men's bodies had been worn out by too much sex, drugs, previous infections, cheeseburger dinners, quiche, and fast-lane life. Their immune systems had simply given up.

This theory touched all the bases: gay men are selfish, upwardly mobile (you have to have a lot of leisure time to get all that sex!), irresponsible, and "dirty." Hell bent on destruction, they don't take the body's signs of minor infection as a hint that perhaps they are overdoing it. Instead, they get shots to conquer VD and caustic carcinogenic potions to wipe out amoebas. The overload theory is an anti-contagion theory: the "public" doesn't live the gay lifestyle and therefore can't get AIDS. In this myth, AIDS is a class illness: people who share certain common characteristics are vulnerable to particular types of disease (in this case sexual practice, but poverty, immigrant status, and race are other qualities that define disease classes). Put another way, types of people get the diseases they deserve. As AIDS turned up in other populations with no clear parallels to the "gay lifestyle," contagion theories gained popularity. (You can almost see it: "Haitians! Intravenous drug users! What next? Say, don't those fags vacation in Haiti and consort with lowlife drug elements?"—and poof! a theory is born.)

Theory two, the Russian roulette theory, posits a "single agent" which is sexually transmitted. Relying on this theory, doctors reasoned that promiscuity leads to inevitable contact with the newly posited deadly agent. Researchers argue that a cluster of gay men early identified as sexual contacts of a single man clued them in to the transmissibility of AIDS. But epidemiology and basic science research reinforce each other's assumptions about who gets a disease, creating an elegant but tautological dance around the central notions of the theory, which in this case are stereotypes of gay men—promiscuity and bizarre practices. Epidemiological models turn out to be wrong as often as they are correct because epidemiology is an inexact, descriptive science. The educated guesses of "disease detectives" are informed by folklore and stereotypes about gay male behavior. In a climate of fear and increased homophobia gay men may well report to epidemiologists the same positive or negative stereotypes they read about themselves, even when their own experience proves otherwise.[5] While multiple partners may well prove to play a role in the transmission of AIDS, scientific reports to date favor a multi-factorial scenario, not a Russian roulette model.

Most researchers are now looking at AIDS in the context of "co-factors"—other elements about the person that may inhibit or assist a single agent. This cluster of co-factors centered around a "prime mover" has the same symbolic impact: any contact with the "AIDS germ" is potentially fatal, legitimizing quarantine, confinement, or legal sanctions for these dangerous sexual activities. Despite the best efforts of some researchers to temper panic, both single agent and co-factor theories are about transmission, and contribute to setting off a contagion and containment panic: identify the germ, the people who have it, and then figure out the most efficient method of staying away from them.

The contemporary notion of dualistically opposed sickness and health blames the sick person for her or his illness: they failed to complete some ritual precaution, like eating well, exercising, or staying out of the way of dirty people. Even the idea that stress is responsible for susceptibility to illness creates a stigma for those who aren't able to cope with the "modern world": sickness becomes a sign that individuals can't manage their responsibilities, or don't express their emotions, and thus make themselves sick.[6] Both types of theory, at least as they become articulated in popular form, "blame the victim."[7]

Because AIDS was early identified as striking a group of people distinguished by their sexuality, the stereotypes and even the research models developed for sexually transmitted diseases kicked into motion. In a society that does not approach homosexuality in the context of a *gay and lesbian culture*, it is problematic to identify sex alone as either the causal factor (overload) or the premiere transmission link (single agent) in the onset of AIDS. AIDS hit the most elaborate of gay male cultures—San Francisco, New York, Los Angeles—and spread to other cities in rough order of size and articulation of gay culture. Although sex, when viewed in the most clinical sense as a special ecosphere for specific agent(s), may indeed prove to be meaningful in AIDS, it is important to consider the implications of using such a volatile and conflated social concept.

Rarely does the medical profession reflect on its own complicity in creating devastating aspects of the AIDS epidemic. Clearly, early detection is important if treatments or preventions are to be developed. Given the rough notions of transmissibility that have informed the "safe sex" guidelines, education is essential. The individuals and groups of people affected by AIDS must therefore have some level of trust in their medical personnel, must believe that the medical industry is concerned about them and their special problems.

Fear of public exposure for being lesbian or gay (VD and now AIDS are mandatorily reportable in most states), an unchallenged belief that one "has to pay the piper," and the relative ease of curing amoebic and bacterial disorders have kept lesbian and gay male, and to a lesser degree straight sexual health care on a curative, rather than a preventative level. Until recently, there has been little emphasis on vaccines or prophylactic aids in the prevention of sexually transmitted diseases (STDs). The solution for those who don't want to catch one is not to have sex outside a monogamous relationship (preferably a heterosexual marriage), medical advice that reinforces traditional social mores.

The opportunistic infections (other than KS and PCP) that accompany AIDS in gay men are precisely those minor infections that have, at least for the last few decades, been a part of the gay male health picture. In AIDS, these irritating ailments become deadly, and even more important to prevent or cure at the earliest possible stage. Yet the historical relationship between lesbians and gay men and their physicians has been hostile and fraught with deception and fear. Gay men especially face ridicule and condemnation for the STDs they may present to their doctors.

STDs serve an important punitive function in this society, even if most require relatively simple, short-term remedies. Doctors serve as the gatekeepers to STD treatment: one must visit this paragon of cleanliness and authority (often in a clinic, where anonymity may be greater) in order to get penicillin or flagyl. Community based STD screening programs have been effectively staffed by volunteers who need much less training. But the social and psychological penalties of "getting caught" with one of these diseases—proof positive of having engaged in illicit sexual activity—are too critical to society's control over sexuality to widely institute these extra-clinical programs.

If the penalties and odds of catching an STD are weighed, the balance tips in favor of waiting for the appearance of clear symptoms, rather than seeking regular preventive screening. Just visiting most clinics for a regular test is a penalty, for it is worse to admit to regularly placing oneself in the position of contracting an STD than somehow to have gotten one "accidentally" (gee, doc, it must have been on the toilet seat). The traditional approach to birth control for women parallels the problem of early screening for VD and education about AIDS prevention: to ask for birth control to avoid unwanted pregnancy (and thereby avoid the later need for an abortion) casts doubt on the morals of the woman seeking contraception, since it is seen as an admission of wanting sex. STDs stand as a reminder that "free sex" is not free, and that non-procreative sex is proscribed.

The terminological shift from "venereal disease" to "sexually transmitted disease" demonstrates the transposition of Victorian sensibility onto the sexual liberation generation. Venereal diseases, while sexually transmitted, were more importantly diseases which appeared on the genitals—vivid symbols of illicit sex. Only in the nineteenth century was it discovered that particular germs were responsible for venereal diseases. But they remained a stigma of improper sexual intercourse. In the 1960s another category of diseases was discovered to be sexually transmitted, although they were not diseases of the genitals. Many of them are amoebic or parasitic diseases that are fairly common among children or in underdeveloped areas. Many are, quite literally, diseases resulting from contact with contaminated feces, directly or in some cases indirectly through eating food that has come in contact with contaminated feces. Despite the common social aversion to feces, it is not the feces themselves that are "dirty," but rather that they provide an amenable environment for various microbes. The relationship of these new sexually transmitted diseases to feces makes them equally offensive markers of illicit sexual activity. Not only are they untidy diseases of the digestive tract, but they are proximate to that most ambivalently regarded point of human anatomy, the asshole. These STDs imply the active involvement of "unnatural acts" in their transmission.

In explaining STDs, and the activities supposedly implicated in AIDS, the generalized conflation of sexual acts and sexual diseases creates innumerable problems. At one time, headlines (at least in the lesbian and gay press) screamed, "Passive anal intercourse linked with AIDS." It wasn't getting fucked, and all that a preference for that position implies, that was the problem. Upon closer reading, one learned that without proper lubrication and care, the fragile anal mucosa could be torn and create a direct pathway for an alleged infectious agent. In a culture that considers men who want to be fucked as true queers, but those who fuck them as just indiscriminate about where they stick their cocks, "passive anal intercourse" at once confirms that real queers are imitation women, and that straight men— who might from time to time stick their manhood in queer holes, but only *dream* of getting fucked—won't get AIDS.

The pervasive and systematic use of penalties like disease and pregnancy (which is treated by doctors as if it were a disease) to inhibit sexual activity is felt by transgressors as a profound and physical terror. The threat of consequences for sex is much more frightening and successful than physical retributions for theft. The idea that you "can't be just a little pregnant" rules out the possibility of calculated risk, and disempowers sexual "transgressors." Larceny is always a calculated risk: the more lucrative, the greater the risk. Sexual acts are socially defined as either perverted or not, even if individual sexual identities allow for much more flexibility. The difficulty which bisexuals have recently experienced in finding a place within the lesbian and gay movement testifies to a failure of even gay liberation rhetoric to make sex situational and not absolute.

The single agent theories escape the problems of levying a consistent penalty by creating the element of chance. If there is a single agent, you could get it from having sex once, or you might never get it. If you are conservative, you will decrease the number of your sex partners. If you are fatalistic, you will just figure that if the germ has your name on it, then it will find you. More so than the overload theories, the single agent theories (whether of germ or sperm) require the afflicted gay man (or pregnant woman) to surrender to doctors and hospitals, since only a doctor is able to see into the tiny, microscopic reaches of the body.

## Lesson two: AIDS and culture

The resistance to understanding and mobilizing to cope with AIDS runs deeper than the structures established to control health care and sex. Illness is not only an individual experience, it is a cultural metaphor. Indeed, next to "the bomb," it may be *the* primary metaphor of the late twentieth century. Although symbolic comparison between the human body and the world is as old as human culture, the contemporary U.S. obsession with disease has turned the metaphor on its head: the notion of the world as sick informs the individual's sense of his or her own illnesses. The post-war idea that communists are a cancer or plague surreptitiously gaining a foothold in the U.S. dramatically recasts individual feelings about being sick, making ill health a form of treason. The "asian flu" becomes a military assault, and citizens are called to "wage war" on disease. And beyond the individual's experience of illness, "disease" becomes a powerful political weapon.

In the late nineteenth century, scientific innovations made "germs" classifiable. The source of at least some diseases became visible through microscopes—special instruments controlled by an increasingly powerful and exclusive profession. "Germs" like spies can sneak unseen into the body, and can only be discovered through special intelligence. The simultaneous discovery of bacteria and the major immigrant movement into the U.S. in the late nineteenth and early twentieth centuries confused the ideas of sickness and foreignness. Even though scientists would argue that it was overcrowding and poor sanitation that led to tragic epidemics in congested urban ghettos, the general population believed that "foreigners" were dirty by nature, and that their dirt (and disease) was proof of their inferiority. Dirt and germs serve an important symbolic role in the social organization of difference. Dirt is chaos, cleanliness order. Disease-stricken people are immoral, healthy people righteous. Zealous turn-of-the-century public health advocates sought to clean up ghettos—attacking real and symbolic dirt. But by the 1920s, the economic cost of purifying urban environments became too great, and public health advocates shifted toward advocating individual rituals of cleansing, such as washing the hands and teeth, in order to ward off disease.

The belief in dirty individuals who leave germs in their wake creates a terror that anyone a little different harbors disease, and has the power to invade the human body. Honest concern about real illness blurs with the need to separate from people feared for racist, sexist, or homophobic reasons. Difference is experienced on a physical level as assault or pollution. On a social scale, the category of "disease" is manipulated to justify genocide, ghettoization, and quarantine: Jews spread the plague, Irish immigrants spread typhoid; prostitutes spread syphilis; drug addicts spread hepatitis; Caribbean boat people spread god-knows-what exotic tropical diseases.

The fear of sexuality parallels the fear of germs. Erotic desires are experienced as a chaos within. People who respond to their sexual desires are labeled obsessed, sick, unable to control themselves. Combined with homophobia, "erotophobia" creates a love that dare not speak its name. Combined with sexism, erotophobia yields desires that dare not speak at all.

In addition to being a sexuality out of control, *homo*sexuality picks the wrong object, and is "unnatural." Homosexuals not only perform disgusting sex acts, but claim sexuality as a celebrated part of identity. As a movement for social change, lesbians and gay men challenge the gender-role structure on which society rests. Homosexuality is "contagious" not just as a method for passing queer germs, but as a model for responding to erotic desires. The social fear that homosexuality will "spread" is always displaced into concern for the "innocent"—children, immature or unwitting adults—never directly for the concerned citizen him/herself.

Racism combined with erotophobia casts Jews, blacks, and latinos as too close to their sexuality, too passionate, out of control. The white racist prohibition against interracial marriage rests on the fear of invasion: the white race will be polluted by black blood.

Only straight, WASP men are believed to be in control of their sexuality, and are given the responsibility for legislating everyone else's through legal and social restrictions and the threat of physical violence. But it is not only straight WASP men who exhibit these germphobic and erotophobic ideas. One of the most difficult obstacles in AIDS organizing has been overcoming preconceptions in the lesbian and gay community about promiscuity and sexual difference, "political" versus "non-political" gays, as if activism somehow protects against catching or transmitting disease.

## The acid test: AIDS organizing—right, left, and queer

If every aspect of the response to AIDS was colored by the history of medicine and science and cultural notions about sex and germs, the manifestations were easier to observe in the far right. Although the right-wing AIDS backlash was about a year late getting started, it built on a decade of anti-gay, anti-sex reactionism. The virulence of the far right, with it's growing structural power, makes it a considerable

political and ideological force in AIDS organizing. Right-wing activists have used AIDS as proof that their pro-family stand is correct,
manipulating fear by using AIDS to defeat lesbian and gay rights bills
and attempting to limit the community's freedom of expression and
right to congregate. Initially, AIDS served only to inflame the recip-
ients of direct mail, no doubt garnering tremendous funds allegedly to
wipe out this "terrible plague." The right expresses little concern for
individual gay men with AIDS (although great concern for "innocent
victims"), and promotes the idea that "selfish" and "sinful" gay men
wander the streets spreading their germs.

The radical left also saw AIDS as an individual problem for a
particular group of gay men who overindulged in that private activity
of sex. In a few cases, leftists brought their political expertise to bear on
AIDS organizing, but there have been virtually no structural or ideological ties between the "political" and "sexual" cultures. Straight
leftists appear comfortable defending the right to engage in private
consensual sexual acts, but perplexed about where to stand on the
public, social consequences of those acts. Unlike the right, the left took
a long time to grasp the idea that because AIDS was connected with
sexuality it made a tremendous potential weapon against lesbian and
gay rights *and* culture. Once each major left media organ had "discovered" this political aspect of AIDS (mostly in the spring of 1983) few
deigned to mention AIDS again until it became apparent that straight
people might also get it.

In the lesbian and gay community, too, there was difficulty in
grasping the magnitude and far-reaching dimensions of AIDS. This
perplexing disease only exacerbated the traditional splits between sex
and politics. This sort of mind/body split appears in complex forms.
Especially for lesbian and gay leftists, maintaining a division between
promiscuity and politics comes in part from the desire to create distance
from death by believing that the men they know will not be at risk for
AIDS. Lesbian and gay activists are not yet free from erotophobia, not
yet convinced by their own rhetoric of sexual liberation. Political
organizing sometimes serves as penance for enjoying the hard-won
sexual freedoms. Political activists' leather fetishes or practice of public
sex are seen as "private," distinct from their politics, which is the more
important aspect of their identity. Lesbian and gay activists of late who
have been "out" as sex radicals find their other political credentials
tainted. In an erotophobic framework, public political activism
becomes a mechanism for integrating private sexuality: mere fucking,
even liberated fucking, is not enough to earn a gay liberation member-
ship card. Activists easily criticize the repression of sexuality, but only

uncomfortably talk of what physical *pleasure* will be gained once sexuality is wrested from the fabric of social penalties and rewards.

The radically different reactions of lesbians and gay men to the appearance of AIDS are related to the broader context of the history of lesbian and gay organizing. Dealing with death and physical attack is nothing new for the gay and lesbian community. Organized and systematic assaults have intruded on this community in the form of police raids on meeting places and queerbashing by gangs of teenagers who are rarely captured and never convicted. Lesbian and gay men are socialized both inside and outside the lesbian and gay community to view their urban subculture as dangerous, unsafe, unprotected from hazards for which mainstream society can erect barriers.

Individually, lesbians and gay men have suffered brutal and sometimes fatal medical and psychological "therapies" designed to change their sexuality. In the mid-eighteenth century, mere masturbation by teenagers could result in castration and clitoridectomy. Homosexuality was warrant for placement in asylums, where surgical and chemical "cures" were employed far into the twentieth century. The 1960s and 1970s saw a decrease in aversion, electroshock, and hormone therapies, but those methods are still elective for people who, if they cannot change their errant sexuality in talking therapies, may opt for more stringent methods. The idea that people can freely choose such harmful therapies for a condition whose only harm is society's displeasure raises grave doubts about the very concept of consent in an oppression-ridden society.

Suicide and self-destructive behavior are other responses to a hostile society. Although the data on suicide and alcohol and drug abuse among lesbians and gay men are equivocal, the idea of participating in a subculture where one is doomed to self-destruction is an important part of the self-image of many gay men and lesbians.[8]

The stress of being a lesbian or gay man is enormous. Worrying about self and friends, and constructing elaborate shields against discovery and persecution occupy a great deal of time for the individual lesbian or gay man. There are virtually no legal or social remedies for the organized and systemic attacks on individuals and on the community by police, ministers, doctors, politicians, and the average citizen with his/her rude comments and methods of home rule that outlaw at least proximate homosexuality.

This sense of constant assault has influenced community and individual responses to AIDS. On one hand, it was a community prepared with strategies hammered out over centuries of oppression to circle the wagons, and count its few friends. The diverse network of social services, political organizations, meeting places, and media built within the lesbian and gay community provided many points of access to exchange information and create a dialogue about response.

But on the other hand, oppression and a decade of organizing had made the community weary, and the need to rise to such a mysterious and deadly assault placed a great demand on a fragile community that is still regrouping after the defeats of the last few years. The lesbian and gay community is undergoing redefinition as the gains that have been made are counted, and the demographics and aspirations of the lesbian and gay population change.

The lesbian and gay community of the early and mid-1980s lacks a sense of shared purpose. The initial radicalism of the 1970s, which inherited its apocalyptic fervor from the 1960s counter-culture, Black Power, and anti-war movements, has seen defection, or at least a tendency toward mainstreaming and reprivatization of sexual identity.

The visibility of the post-Stonewall movement led the lesbian and gay left toward coalition-building with other progressive movements. On the strength of its history, lesbian and gay liberation fought its way into the "rainbow coalition." This is a major victory: liberals and leftists acknowledge the minority status of lesbians and gay men, even if they only dimly understand the true meaning of lesbian and gay liberation.

Other lesbian and gay men, especially those with more economic power, have created successful urban ghettos where it is easier to be lesbian or gay than ever before. But the establishment of viable economic communities too often comes at the cost of displacing other minority communities, as "gaylining" replaces redlining. The gay ghetto wields economic and political power only in relation to competing disenfranchised groups, and the very "clone revolution" that confirms the existence of a visible gay male community runs at odds with the rainbow coalition's attempts to create lasting political bonds with other minorities.

Both trends contribute to the evolution of the lesbian and gay community in building community centers, political and religious organizations, bars, restaurants, clothing styles, and sexual possibilities. And there are people who live in both arenas, promoting a dialogue between these two forms of gay and lesbian liberation. But there is a lack of common language and shared project. When AIDS hit, the former "activists" were involved in the more comprehensive issues of coalition-building, while the "clones," who would appear to be first and hardest hit by AIDS, were busy consolidating ghetto life, without the benefit of the organizational strategies and ideology that had won a modicum of rights and political clout. The initial reaction of the urban clones was that AIDS was an individual problem which required group support and a group solution. But they soon encountered the systemic complexities: homophobia, racism, and sexism set up blocks at every turn.

The AIDS organizing within the lesbian and gay community has grown into a curious mix of radical and traditional politics involving education, support, direct action, and coalition-building. But AIDS organizing, it was soon discovered, is significantly different from other projects. There are the usual conflicts about structure and process, about politics and support. But at no other time had I been involved in a project where one day I would learn that someone with whom I had planned meetings or argued a political point was suddenly, and unalterably, "one of them." A person with AIDS. One day we were working together as equals, and the next a sentence of finitude created an unbridgeable gulf. Being involved in AIDS organizing means agreeing to build community with people who may be dead in two months. And there is no way to know who will be next.

Of course, there are parallel tragedies in other types of organizing. People die unexpectedly, and they die as a direct result of racism, sexism, and homophobia. But in AIDS organizing, death circles around at shortening intervals. It is not unexpected, even if it is always a shock, and it is rarely sudden. Death is a daily part of the organizing. Dealing with AIDS on any level—political, support, individual, as a journalist—means dealing with death as part of the whole fabric of organizing.

Yet, these deaths feel different from ones that come as a result of racist or homophobic murders, or sexist mismanagement of abortion. AIDS is an extreme and more directed form of social violence that controls groups of people by saying, "You asked for it"—by what you wore, where you went, or in this case by whom you chose to love. AIDS deaths are blamed on the dying, and those who are close to them: the individual friends and the entire lesbian and gay community. AIDS falls neatly on the extreme end of the sex punishment continuum: masturbation will give you hairy palms; premarital sex, pregnancy; extramarital sex, VD; gay sex, death. For gay men there is a constant, nagging tension that you got or will get AIDS from someone you love. Or that you will infect an "innocent" trick, or a favorite friend. Regardless of the medical facts—which may in time show which other significant factors like genes, prior disease history, or physical environment are essential in the AIDS picture—there is an inescapable feeling that sex, the thing which to some important degree defines gay identity and community, is the cause of the killing. It is extremely difficult to escape this sex-negative ethos when people are dying of AIDS every day. It heightens a diffuse anger that lesbian and gay men carry as a minority under attack. Even the ability to make sense of AIDS in a good, gay liberation perspective does not wipe away the anguish and shattering sense of defeat felt each time another person is diagnosed with AIDS, each time another person confronts the additional prejudice of living with AIDS, each time friends and community must face the final tragedy of another life ended by AIDS. The caseload numbers tell only the smallest, least personal aspects of AIDS, but like the body count litany that brought home the agony of the Vietnam war, they serve as impressive, abstract reminders that AIDS has not, and in a very real sense, will never go away.

The intense ambivalence and fears about both sexuality and disease are too overpowering to permit much rational discourse on the politics of sex and germs. Yet this dimension, as well as an understanding of the immediate tragedy, is essential to successfully connect individual experiences with the social and political structures that impede attempts to cope with AIDS at every level.

The failure to relate AIDS to the historical context of modern medicine, to past lesbian and gay liberation and progressive efforts, has resulted in something much less than the broad and united front necessary for an effective response to AIDS. Neither the majority of veteran gay/lesbian activists, the women's movement, nor the left has lent much assistance to the relatively new AIDS activists. The result has been a perpetuation of some of the classic forms of oppression within AIDS organizing, as well as a persistent homophobia, erotophobia, and basic misunderstanding of the magnitude of AIDS outside the organizing effort.[9] To those outside AIDS organizing, AIDS continues to be viewed primarily as a single issue. To those inside, the range and complexity of issues tapped seem almost impossible to combat. People involved in AIDS organizing have learned quickly the lessons of lesbian and gay organizing, anti-sexist and anti-racist work, but without benefit of veterans who might have suggested courses of action that would have avoided reinventing the political wheel.

The divisions within the gay and lesbian community (and to a great extent outside it) that have prohibited a unified response to AIDS rest on unresolved political questions, not the least of which are the relationships between sex and sexual liberation, between sexual liberation and other areas of liberation.

AIDS organizing *could* provide a context for a discussion of sexuality in the broader gay and lesbian movement. But as long as the discussion of the meaning of sex is confined to those who fear contracting a deadly disease, then past sex-negative patterns will be repeated: good sex doesn't result in disease, but disease proves the existence of bad sex.

The challenge of AIDS organizing for progressive movements is to create a new and more comprehensive understanding of sexuality and its control, and a reintegration of the body into political discourse. The lesson learned daily in AIDS is that the state regulates our bodies through control of sexuality and health. A progressive agenda that addresses the many aspects of oppression possible in this nexus of sexuality and health could create new possibilities for coalition across many traditional areas of political work—race, class, sex, creative living.

AIDS seems to be making exploratory forays into the "mainstream," affecting the people who until recently did not live under the fear of this little-understood new disease. But equally important is the political testing of waters: the new conservatism is using AIDS to see just how far it can go in reinstating controls over the body only briefly jarred loose by the new left, black civil rights, women's liberation, and gay liberation movements. The test of these groups' commitment to broad social liberation will be found in the total response to AIDS. The gay and lesbian community will certainly be scrutinized for its response to AIDS. But other progressive movements, too, will be asked the question: "What was your response when AIDS and AIDS-phobia ran wild through the gay, Haitian, IV-drug, and prostitute communities?"

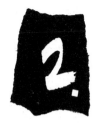

# They Said It Couldn't Happen

According to popular wisdom, an epidemic like AIDS should not have been possible. Modern medicine has conquered communicable disease. The epidemics faced in recent history have been virtually wiped out. Polio, cholera, and bubonic plague occur only in isolated cases. The traditional venereal diseases, childhood illnesses, and even influenza are readily identifiable and quickly cured with minimal long-term effect on the patient. The twentieth-century sensibility of U.S. superpower strength admits no plagues, no deadly communicable diseases of unknown origin. In the pantheon of dreaded illness, only cancer remains to be conquered. And yet, the relatively disease-free U.S. citizen is obsessed with disease, engendering a whole field of medical journalism to provide up-to-date information. Disease reportage creates its market by stoking the residual fears of massive onslaughts by disease and then calming the reader with incomprehensible "discoveries" that will erect an even greater barrier against germs. The professionalization of modern medicine, medical journalism, and medicine-related law has produced a vast self-referential collection of medical understandings and misunderstandings.

If the occasional appearance of a Legionnaire's disease or toxic shock syndrome challenges the belief in immunity from disastrous mystery diseases, the public is rapidly consoled by the discovery that these new plagues are merely variants of already conquered germs. These medical dramas serve to reinforce the rule: disease has been conquered; the public witnesses this miracle in its own lifetime.

Chapter 5 will trace the history of U.S. medical professionals' rise to power, examining the impact of the domestication of germs on the social understanding of disease. But a peculiar and scientifically incorrect *cultural* concept should be noted here: the world is divided into us and germs. In reality, many "germs" live happily and even helpfully in and on the human body, and at least some illnesses result from the mislocation of these happy germs in the wrong part of the body. Rarely is the body conceptualized as a balanced world of microscopic elements that keep each other in check. This entrenched concept opposing "us" and "germs" underlies the medical and symbolic understanding of AIDS, a phenomenon where the organisms which usually present no major problem become deadly in the person whose underlying AIDS prevents her or him from launching a defense.

From a medical standpoint, the traditional "germs" *have* been conquered, and even the particular "germs" which cause illness in the person with AIDS (the so-called opportunistic infections) could be "cured" under normal circumstances. But people with AIDS cannot fully recover because treatments are predicated on immune system functions which no longer exist in those patients. AIDS is a profound assault on the complacent U.S. view of disease: at the very moment in history when disease was declared conquered, a new syndrome removed the very elements within the body that had once cooperated with the doctor's treatment.

Despite qualitative and quantitative improvements in health care delivery, people die for no apparent reason every day. There continue to be an estimated 50,000 to 70,000 cases of some form of Legionnaire's disease, with as many as 3,000 deaths annually, and thirty to thirty-five toxic shock syndrome cases each month, with a 3 percent death rate. There are even occasional bubonic plague deaths and mini-epidemics of cholera.[1]

Diseases in the developed world rarely achieve the epidemic proportions of plagues and poxes of the past. Death from disease has not been conquered, even if the incidence has decreased. There is a mystique surrounding who gets a disease and who does not, a phenomenon which is usually explained by associating a particular disease with traits of some group of people. As rampant disease is conquered, and the middle class U.S. citizen has less contact with disease, it becomes even easier to associate new diseases with particular distant groups of people. The organization of medical surveillance, media coverage, and patterns of medical delivery lend credence to this superstitious view of the genesis of disease.

First, new or revived diseases always appear to strike in one place or to affect one group of people first. Often, the disease actually does strike in this localized or population-specific fashion. Legionnaire's disease achieved media prominence when it hit an identifiable group at a single location, even though there were numerous less clear-cut cases. Toxic shock syndrome, an infection by a known bacteria, was identified in relation to a defined population of women who used particular brands of tampons. In the case of AIDS, clusters of like cases triggered medical attention. A series of individual cases in small towns would not have come to public attention as quickly as half a dozen cases of rare pneumonia in Los Angeles and another half dozen cancer cases in New York, all among identifiably gay urban men.

Second, both the real distance and media-portrayed distance from disease mean that new diseases are experienced as existing "out there" among some other group of people, unless they are "here" among one's own community. The "self" and "other" labeling of disease is partly due to media coverage which reports on medical phenomena that the general public would not otherwise encounter. In AIDS, the media both created the "gay plague" mentality but also educated doctors and at-risk people all over the world about the possibility of encountering AIDS.

Finally, access to medical care and attention to disease have been greatest for middle-class families living close to cities. The diseases conquered first were those affecting "the average person"; diseases that continue to affect urban poor, gay men, IV drug users, hemophiliacs, or prostitutes are still not well-addressed. Access to services for illness related to poverty or sexuality is limited by financial, cultural, and logistical barriers, and through stigmatization for seeking care. In addition, medical problems that are built into the structure of modern medicine go unreported. As many transfused patients contract non-A, non-B hepatitis as transfusion-associated AIDS; indeed, as many die because clerical errors in labeling resulted in patients receiving the wrong unit of blood.[2]

The increasingly powerful media have played an important role in creating the false sense that the U.S. is free from disease. Sensational and overly macroscopic views of scientific events misinterpret the microscopic and tentative work of medical researchers. Some doctors and researchers seem to revel in the media attention, carelessly reporting equivocal findings which the competitive media all too happily misreport as cures. They seem to take a supply-side view of medical information: giving people theories as facts, discoveries as breakthroughs, makes them feel better and ends the epidemic through sheer force of will. Sensationalism, this school of information dissemination implies, will scare the faggots out of having sex. But the isolation of an alleged etiologic agent is only a preliminary step toward developing a vaccine, and a vaccine will not help those already exposed to the presumed virus, who need treatment to combat AIDS and other long-term effects. Media terrorism often serves to make the lesbian and gay community skeptical about any of the information at all.

The over 12,000 people who have AIDS are not fooled by this kind of magic trick, and the demand for accurate reporting of medical information is part of their fight for life. The media compete for viewers and readers, with a premium on cataclysms that attract attention, not on solutions which are usually painstaking and uninteresting. The sudden appearance of disease is reported, and sometimes the cure sees its way into print if it is bizarre or dramatic, or saves babies. Epidemics are sexy. Cures can be made sexy by inflating the role of that god, science. Real people with real diseases are too boring for the media to incorporate into ongoing reporting, unless these individuals can be depicted as exotic or pathetic victims. The costs to a community, especially to an already stigmatized community, are ignored. Even reports like the June 1985 *Life* magazine cover story, "Now No One is Safe," confirm the otherness of AIDS: titillated by the possibility of a deadly mystery disease, readers eventually learn that they will not encounter AIDS unless they *become like* those in risk groups.

## AIDS invades the American consciousness

The first AIDS cases were reported in 1981, although retrospective analysis of unexplained deaths identified cases dating back to the late 1970s. The medical establishment first took note of this burgeoning syndrome in two separate collections of cases—one in Los Angeles, one in New York. The Centers for Disease Control became aware of this perplexing constellation of extreme immune system failures in the winter of 1980 and made preparations to publish reports in the spring and summer of 1981. At first, the cases seemed dissimilar, except for the "and by the way" notation by the reporting clinicians that the patients were young, "previously healthy," gay men.[3] The six cases were deaths due to *pneumocistis carinii*, a very rare pneumonia previously seen only in patients whose immune systems had been debilitated by chronic severe illness or as a result of some kinds of dramatic therapies. The Los Angeles gay men had rapidly deteriorated from good health, and died of PCP suddenly.

The New York cases showed virulent Kaposi's sarcoma, a usually slow cancer appearing as skin lesions. Kaposi's sarcoma had been identified in the 1800s and occurred mainly in elderly Italian or Ashkenazi Jewish men. In these classic cases of KS, the lesions began on the lower extremities and only after many years affected internal organs. Most of these people died of other causes. The new KS cases, however, showed early appearance on the trunk and neck, with rapid spread to internal organs. This virulent new KS was fatal in cases where internal spread was rapid.

The early identification of AIDS with the at-risk gay population set the tone for media coverage, delivery of medical care, and even for research. The media continued to link the illness with irresponsibility and sex, blaming gays for their illness. Hemophiliacs, transfusion cases, children, and wives of men with AIDS who came down with the syndrome were consistently called "innocent victims," who through no fault of their own were standing in the path of a dread disease. The continuing media implication is that AIDS is spread by a much less than innocent population—gay men (picture a drooling pervert), IV drug users (picture the local junkie), Haitians (picture a black bagperson), and finally by prostitutes. These are the images conjured up by the fits and starts of mass media AIDS coverage, manipulated to terrify middle America and to dishearten those in risk groups by adding discrimination to the threat of illness.

The particular problems of hemophiliacs have been largely ignored. Although included as "innocent victims" in media accounts, AIDS has compounded the stigmatization these men face. Although "innocent" of presumed sexual difference, the myths about hemophilia and taboo links with blood and bleeding make AIDS among hemophiliacs not quite "clean" and best kept hidden. One hemophiliac describes the growing fear that hemophiliacs are dangerous to employ or to have in schools as "hemophobia," and speaks wryly of coming out of the "clot closet." AIDS hit at a time when hemophiliacs, often socialized to feel that they couldn't lead a "normal life" and stereotyped as weak men, were becoming more open about their special medical condition and were finally finding social acceptance. As a medical syndrome, hemophilia, like AIDS, renders those affected uninsurable. Hemophiliacs are now facing job discrimination due to the belief that they harbor AIDS, and the ludicrous fear that they will bleed all over everyone at work.

The medical delivery system was also hit hard by the appearance of AIDS. Although not a single health care worker has come down with AIDS through casual contact with AIDS patients, and studies of needlestick accidents reveal no transmission of HTLV-III/LAV, ambulance attendants, dentists, nurses, even doctors have refused to treat

AIDS patients.[4] San Francisco issued surgical masks and gloves to police who feared they would catch AIDS while arresting gay men. In prison AIDS cases, sick inmates have been transferred or isolated, their effects burned, and their cells scrubbed. One man, angered by his treatment at a prestigious hospital, put a pink triangle on his hospital room door and marked it "AIDS Camp," a reference to homosexual prisoners in Nazi concentration camps, who were required to wear a pink triangle.

### It's all in the name

Diseases and syndromes are named in a number of ways. Well-known traditional diseases often retain their colloquial names—like the cold. Other diseases may be renamed after their etiological agent—as in strep throat, named for the streptococcus bacteria—or for the person who defines the distinctive qualities of the disease—as with Kaposi's sarcoma, named for the German scientist who in 1864 described and researched this particular type of tumor, formed in connective tissue (rather than in covering tissue, tumors called carcinomas).

Sometimes new diseases are named for the group of people they originally strike. The Centers for Disease Control often use this terminology until they are able to discover whether a new or newly epidemic disease is actually some known disease in a new or different form. Legionnaire's disease was named after its most publicized hosts, even though it could have received the name of its bacterial cause, which has now been identified in at least seven varieties.

AIDS was originally named GRID—Gay-Related Immune Deficiency—until gay activists objected to naming what was then an unresearched syndrome after an already stigmatized group. When no immediate cause could be identified for the constellation of fatal illnesses in a diverse set of groups, scientists shifted to Acquired Immune Deficiency Syndrome, to distinguish it from other known immunodeficiency problems related to the very young, the very old, or people who had experienced major bodily trauma. (Children do not develop a fully active immune system until they are about two, and the elderly often experience greater susceptibility to disease, especially if they are taking drugs for other problems associated with aging.)

AIDS was first defined by the CDC as a syndrome striking previously healthy people between the ages of fifteen and sixty, in which infections that are not usually fatal lead to severe illness progressing to death. The age range has been extended in cases where it is clear that a child or person over sixty fits into a risk group and does not have another underlying problem, or can be shown through experimental tests to have markers of AIDS. The key feature of AIDS is an acute depression of the immune system with no classic explanation. Much remains unknown about immune function in general. Immune system functioning has not been routinely tested, and at this point, AIDS is only evident when a secondary infection appears. Less dramatic symptoms such as wasting, persistently swollen lymph nodes, night sweats, persistent fevers, are now classified variously as persistent generalized lymphadenopathy, pre-AIDS, lesser AIDS, AIDS prodrome, or most commonly, AIDS-Related Complex, or ARC. Little is known about how many of these people will progress to full-blown AIDS, nor is there any understanding of why some people progress to full-blown AIDS and others do not. Although several types of infection endemic to gay men are opportunistic infections in AIDS, the exact role of homosexuality or homosexual practice in AIDS remains unknown.

The CDC, then, defines a disease in a way that facilitates quick identification of likely cases, and points toward the etiology and epidemiology of the new illness. Diseases are named for the convenience of the researchers and doctors, with little concern for the effect of the naming on the populations affected. With the discovery of HTLV-III/LAV, some researchers have moved toward renaming AIDS "HTLV-III disease."

## A lesson in geometry

AIDS cases grew at a phenomenal rate. Doctors all over the U.S. and around the world read about AIDS in the *Morbidity and Mortality Weekly Report*, or in mainstream media reports, and submitted cases of their own. A controversial decision by Dr. Edward Brandt, head of the National Institute of Health until late 1984, pressured medical journals to expedite publication of AIDS-related research, opening the floodgate for mangled press accounts but permitting some researchers to publish and apply for research monies more quickly.[5]

In 1983 there was confusion about the number of AIDS cases. The CDC was slow to evaluate and count submitted cases, and AIDS organizations saw many extremely sick people who lacked a CDC criterion. AIDS groups knew of people who were denied an AIDS diagnosis up until their death, thereby disqualifying them for Social Security benefits and contributing to underestimation of the crisis's impact.

The CDC resolved to count cases more quickly, but the major AIDS groups kept their own counts of cases submitted and cases accepted. Many people believe that because of under reporting due to ignorance or prejudice in non-urban areas, there may be many more cases of AIDS than have been reported. Anecdotal evidence in non-gay at-risk populations suggests that many cases go unreported here as well (although doctors are required to report AIDS in many states, they do not always do so, deferring to patients who do not want their diagnosis known). Because of the long and variable incubation period, the figures will continue to swing upward at a rapid rate. In initial years of AIDS incidence in a location, new cases increase at a geometric rate, but later the percentage increase of new cases stays the same. The two cities with the largest number of AIDS cases—San Francisco and New York—have leveled off in their *rate* of increase, but the smaller cities and towns are experiencing the geometric increase. Boston, for example, which saw only about five cases during the time New York was first experiencing the doubling phenomenon (1982), saw forty cases in the fall of 1983, but had 180 cases by the fall of 1984, with a new case every thirty-six hours at the end of the year, and a case per day by late summer 1985. New Hampshire and Vermont in the fall of 1984 were seeing the caseload that Massachusetts had seen in 1982. Pittsburgh at the end of 1984 began to resemble Boston in 1983. With no solid clues to transmissibility, and great misunderstanding within most of the medical establishment about gay sexual practices, including urban/rural differences, the duration of cyclic explosion in specific areas is speculative.

AIDS—especially in the gay male populations—strikes a set of sub-communities that are bound together by cultural similarities and some migration. It resembles classic epidemics with multiple centers related to shipping patterns which provided a mobile human vector of transmission. As in many epidemics of the past, community composition and mobility may provide a key to understanding. Each city where AIDS appears has different gay community patterns and histories, sexual mores, and even sexual practices, with differing levels of gay health care and possibly different opportunistic disease pools which affect the secondary disease patterns in AIDS. The regional differences in how AIDS is expressed may reveal unexpected information, as will comparing morbidity and mortality differences nationally and internationally in the various at-risk groups.

Scientists must reorient their assumptions that gay men represent a homogeneous population. Medical researchers usually look for similarities: early assumptions about the at-risk groups, such as use of certain drugs, promiscuity, certain sexual practices, must be critically examined since they mimic traditional prejudices and may obscure other factors not stereotypically associated with the at-risk groups. Serious attention to the presumed heterosexual transmission of AIDS in African cases and in female partners of men with or at risk for AIDS in the U.S., as well as a closer examination of possible co-factors that are population-specific, will help right the skewed research models that are too heavily predicated on social stereotypes.

## A diverse disease

It is difficult to get a complete sense of the symptoms of AIDS from any single case, so diverse and non-specific is the range of symptoms. The aggregate of possible symptoms suggests the complexity of clinical AIDS, but the profile created by this summary definition of risk factors and symptoms is too often read back as the *typical* case. Many people fall outside of this summary definition, which can mask the reality of their medical and social problems.

AIDS and related disorders have a broad clinical spectrum from frank AIDS to ARC and possible chronic complications. The diversity of this new illness constellation creates enormous social and political problems, reflected in the wide range of medical and organizational efforts launched to cope with the crisis. People with AIDS progress through their illness at vastly different rates and with a wide range of comfort and ability to continue their daily activities. Some people die suddenly and are only retrospectively diagnosed with AIDS. A person with opportunistic infections may be in and out of treatment for several years with successful recovery from particular episodes. But the periods out of the hospital are shorter and shorter until the person finally cannot recover. Some patients with KS only have shown a remarkable ability to control the spread of lesions and feel relatively well. But the lesions may precipitously spread to internal organs, or another opportunistic infection may tip the balance, causing an individual who was feeling well to require sudden hospitalization and even die.

Those providing services, support, and friendship to people with AIDS are in a totally unpredictable situation, resulting in great stress and uncertainty for people with AIDS and their support workers. Organizations have developed flexible programs in order to cope with these rapidly changing and widely differing circumstances. As more people are diagnosed with AIDS and chronic AIDS-related problems are identified, organizers find themselves in the category of "the sick." Constantly dealing with sickness and death makes AIDS organizing depressing, but forces those involved to confront their carefully constructed defense mechanisms. There is always a possible person with AIDS on every steering committee, even when organizers feel that the people they are trying to help are "out there." AIDS groups must build in a support system for the organizers. As more people with AIDS join AIDS organizations, and as more people in AIDS organizations get AIDS, roles are constantly challenged. With evolving definitions of AIDS and ARC—and the new HTLV-III/LAV antibody test identifies an asymptomatic but anti-positive group—new levels of support and educational efforts are needed.

The broad definition of symptoms is not unusual for a new disease or syndrome. Epidemiological history is full of stories of apparent new diseases which were attributed with nearly every symptom in the book. Later, as more was known about the difference between one disease and its near relatives, symptoms took on a more definitive hue. Popular recountings of "disease detectives" reveal the relationships between prior knowledge and technology and concepts of new diseases. Thus, for example, two diseases might be considered the same until a new drug is developed which combats one disease, but not the other. The interplay between epidemiology and basic research is important, since they work together in an often tautological fashion to create new definitions of particular diseases in order to study and to treat them.

Although the Western categories of disease seem logical and objectively structured, they are pragmatic, dependent on the range of therapies and technologies available. For example, the symptoms of AIDS are identical to malaise, flus, or mild infections. The diffuse symptoms suggest AIDS only when they are not attributable or treatable, or when definite secondary infections show that an individual has lost the ability to restore a healthy balance on their own. Those who perceive themselves to be at risk scrutinize each ache or sleepless night. Hotlines receive innumerable calls from people who are not at risk, but are concerned about symptoms they believe are related to improbable contact with an at-risk person. The public's confusion about the signs and symptoms of AIDS stems from historical shifts in the popular understanding of disease, a topic which will be explored at greater length in Chapter 5.

A final irony of symptomatology triggered the political crisis surrounding AIDS. In most diseases, some group of people is thought to be particularly susceptible, or *at risk* for the disease. For example, children are particularly at risk for mumps or measles, older people for influenza's more dramatic consequences. With AIDS, however, the notion of being at risk soon slid over into being a symptom. Thus, being homosexual somehow became a symptom of AIDS in the public eye, and having AIDS became a sign of being homosexual.

# The Search for a Magic Bullet

The discovery of a presumed "AIDS virus," as HTLV-III/LAV would soon be known, was leaked to the press and gay leaders, making its official appearance on April 23, 1984. The most immediate effect of this announcement was to expose the nearly one-year blackout on AIDS coverage. Following the initial blitz of mainstream media attention during the summer and fall of 1983, AIDS had more or less dropped out of sight in the straight press. Nearly every major U.S. magazine and many influential European journals had run a story on AIDS, with angles ranging from personal tragedy to political impact. But none had really grasped the extent of the crisis on a sizable and increasingly visible U.S. lesbian and gay community, nor had they understood the politics of the disease except in the most gross financial terms. AIDS was striking gay male baby-boomers—a generation whose consciousness had been shaped by the cynicism of an "America" lost to Vietnam and Watergate, and whose political activism had fused counter-cultural values with civil rights assimilation. No one predicted the impact of a controversial and deadly disease on this particular community of men. With no cures or discoveries, the straight media was unable to come up with an angle that justified waving the gay male world before the averted eyes of the average citizen. As a community hurt by the double-edged sword of invisibility and gross stereotype, gay and lesbian organizations have become expert at locking horns with the media. Some newspapers had become AIDS-shy: they had been harshly criticized for sensational or insensitive AIDS coverage, and solved the problem by avoiding any coverage at all.

The discovery of HTLV-III caught the liberal media off guard. The *New York Times* and *Boston Globe* had been none too easy on the Reagan administration, yet here was the Secretary of Health and Human Services announcing a breakthrough in the "gay plague"!

The situation was complicated: U.S. scientists were busy tripping over each other either to claim credit for the breakthrough or to give it away to the French, who had one year earlier discovered what was believed by many scientists to be the same virus. It took almost a week before there was a coherent explanation of exactly *what* had been discovered, and still longer before the significance of the discovery could be assessed.

Several highly respected newspapers ran equivocal headlines above say-nothing stories. On April 19, for example, the *Boston Globe* reported: "Virus believed to cause AIDS is reportedly identified." And three days later: "US to identify virus as AIDS cause." After Secretary of Health and Human Services Margaret Heckler's press conference on April 23, they said only, "Virus tied to AIDS is identified, doctor says."

It was not until Sunday the 24th that the *New York Times* science section deigned to explain in detail what the scientific part of the fuss was about: the development by Dr. Robert Gallo of the National Institute of Health's National Cancer Institute, in Bethesda, Maryland, of a special super cell that could harbor human T-lymphotropic virus (HTLV-III) long enough to cultivate that virus in large quantities. HTLV-III, Gallo believes, is the primary cause of AIDS.

Gallo's development was important because scientists need to produce sufficient quantities of suspect viruses in order to duplicate in the laboratory the natural progression of viral disease in humans. Ultimately, they must duplicate the illness in laboratory animals in order to develop and test a vaccine.

The difference between finding a virus and figuring out how to mass produce it is both scientifically and professionally significant for competitive researchers. Inventing tools and techniques reeks of manufacturing, while the discovery of a new source of evil for the boys in white to gun down is heroic. Discovery of both the virus and the technique confers godlike status. That is exactly what Gallo claimed to have done.

There was, however, one hitch. The Institute Pasteur in Paris had already announced, almost a year before, that it had isolated lymphadenopathy associated virus (LAV), which their studies indicated as the likely cause of AIDS. In addition, a British laboratory had identified

AIDS related virus (ARV), also believed to be the etiological AIDS agent, and a Berkeley, California lab would soon announce the cultivation of what might prove to be the same virus. Whether these viruses were the same, related viruses, or variants of a single virus remained to be tested, although the enthusiasm for cross checking the various isolates dwindled quickly.

## Living with HTLV-III

The discovery of HTLV-III quickly proved to be more of a burden than a sign of hope for a panic-stricken lesbian and gay community. Gallo seemed—at least to gay media writers and editors—to be more interested in his career than in helping people who were trying to cope with AIDS. Although he feels he has been unfairly attacked, what he says does little to make the lesbian and gay community feel comfortable with him. James D'Eramo, Ph.D., a medical writer for the New York *Native*, interviewed Gallo in the summer of 1984. Gallo revealed his insensitivity with statements in that interview that he had "heard that there are some [gay men] who are so sexually driven that they act like alcoholics." He added doom to insult when he said that although he was not a clinical doctor (and here his lack of knowledge of gay men and their lifestyles and sexual identity is most glaring), "What I believe is far more cautious than avoiding certain sexual practices. I would advocate sexual abstinence until this problem is solved. It may be a while, it may be a lifetime. I'm sorry, I'm doing my best."[1]

But it is not only the lesbian and gay community that seems to resent Gallo's expansive and insistent forays into the press. The Centers for Disease Control in Atlanta, the other major U.S. government research facility investigating AIDS, consistently throughout the spring 1984 media blitz credited the French with the discovery of the likely agent implicated in the etiology of AIDS. Just a few days before Margaret Heckler claimed the discovery for the U.S., Mason would budge only enough to congratulate Gallo on the development of a new method for producing large quantities of HTLV-III in the laboratory. James O. Mason, head of the CDC, told the *New York Times* that the French had isolated the virus first. There were hints in the same *New York Times* article that the NIH had been less than vigorous in pursuing the French LAV lead, while Gallo blamed the communication gap on laboratory techniques and the Institute Pasteur's lack of enthusiasm.[2] Two *Boston Globe* articles in June 1984 turned the apparent inter-agency conflict into a "Hollywood style" race to the finish between the French and U.S. scientists.

Quickly, five companies were granted permits to develop an HTLV-III test kit, contingent on later FDA approval. A sixth company announced in early July that they would pursue a LAV test with the Institute Pasteur. This company claims that it has priority over the patented cell line, since the Institute Pasteur applied for worldwide patent rights in September of 1983, while Gallo's work was not patented until the spring of 1984. According to the *Wall Street Journal*, the tests would find a $100 million market once developed.[3]

Disaffected lesbian and gay activists and the U.S. doctors who disagreed either in substance or in tone with Gallo's research weren't the only people to question the significance and media attention given to the HTLV-III discovery. Dr. Jan van Wigngaarden, the Dutch AIDS coordinator, said that he did not think Gallo had sufficient proof for his assertions about the workings of the HTLV-III virus in AIDS, and he questioned the use of a "blood test" which can neither prove the existence of AIDS nor predict who will get AIDS and who will not. D'Eramo reported in the *Native* that the "Dutch intimated that the announcement of Gallo's findings by Secretary of Health Margaret Heckler could be viewed as a publicity maneuver for the Reagan re-election campaign."[4]

HTLV-III became a hot topic in a community becoming rapidly disillusioned with the power of modern medicine to cure. The anxious at-risk groups needed to believe that doctors, and by extension medical researchers, were acting in their best interests, but medicine and medical research are major industries, motivated by a desire for prestige and money. The researcher is given grants based on her or his past work; the more impressive it has been, the more likely is receipt of further funding. And the various drug and chemical companies, closely connected with at least some of the top researchers in every field, are waiting in the wings with their patent lawyers.

Medical and scientific discoveries do not end up in the public domain. Mere mortals benefit from these rarefied bits of genius only when they trickle down into actual drugs and tests, all at a hefty cost to the consumer. A lot of money and probably a Nobel prize are at stake in the AIDS Olympics, and those who will benefit first and most handsomely will not be those who have the disease. Despite the sweeping claims of Heckler and Gallo, most doctors believe it is unlikely that a vaccine will be widely available soon, if it is possible to develop one at all. It took nearly ten years to get hepatitis B vaccine, and there is still no vaccine for toxic shock, a much less complex syndrome than the elusive AIDS. Some researchers believe that the AIDS virus is rapidly mutating, making it nearly impossible to develop a continuously effective vaccine.[5]

Although a great deal of other important research was underway, however, the media picked up on HTLV-III and then rode it into the ground, quickly shifting from "the possible AIDS agent" to calling HTLV-III the "AIDS virus." Why this emphasis on virus hunting? The tipoff was emblazoned across the full-color *USA Today* of April 24, 1984: "AIDS test to cut risk in transfusions." A subtle mix of campaign hype and the need to create a boundary between the groups at risk for AIDS and the general population found the hypothetical HTLV-III antibody test a convenient symbol with which to reassure the increasingly nervous "general public." A quick and easy "safe blood test" to protect "innocent victims" makes much better press than updates on the trial measures to alleviate the symptoms of the small minority of people who already have AIDS. The blood test itself is not all it's cracked up to be, even though United Airlines and other employers have sought to use it as a requirement for employment (see Chapter 6). The assays for HTLV-III actually look for *antibody* to the virus, since the virus itself is concealed within a subset of cells in the immune system and difficult to test for. The assays developed to date produce false positives and false negatives. While this is true of any test, the high stakes of AIDS and lack of secondary diagnostic tools make this test particularly insidious. No one knows whether presence of the antibody (or even the virus) indicates communicability or whether there is a chronic carrier state, as with hepatitis B.

## HTLV-III: the key to the discrimination lock

The most problematic aspect of hyping HTLV-III is its potential social and political impact. Finding an agent highly correlated with AIDS, if for unclear reasons, is a critical step. In a sense, the discovery of HTLV-III recapitulated the course of more general AIDS hysteria; there was a new name, and the new possibility of more clearly defining the "other," those people who were infected. The hysteria of the "casual contact" scare of late 1983 kicked back into motion. The casual contact papers, published in *The New England Journal of Medicine*, were inaccurately reported in the press as "proof" that AIDS could be spread through "household" contact, although the major dailies backed off from that story in their second editions. But the possibility that AIDS might spread suddenly and rapidly provoked an unknown number of public health departments to dust off quarantine statutes. Astonished lesbian and gay activists quickly discovered that public health departments already had the power to lock up everyone sus-pected of having or getting AIDS; all they needed was some mechanism by which to decide exactly whom to lock up.

HTLV-III seemed to provide that key. The more savvy and media-burnt researchers urged caution in interpreting HTLV-III find-ings, but the media had already blown the discovery's immediate impact far out of proportion. The wildly careening "AIDS virus" breakthrough dwarfed its detractors and other research that pointed in different or more cautious directions.

## HTLV-III testing: no respite from uncertainty

Since the beginning of the AIDS epidemic, one group of people after another experienced the chilling sense of uncertainty brought on by being identified as at risk for the syndrome that has no known cause, and no clear reason for choosing one person or group over another. For a long time, gay men bemoaned the lack of a test or marker for AIDS, feeling that if someone could tell them whether they had it or not they could at least get on with reshaping the rest of their lives. As soon as ARC was identified a new category of uncertainty was created. Those staffing hotlines and working with support or information groups quickly learned that these men and women were psychologically more fragile than those who had received a certain diagnosis of AIDS. For all of the tragedy, bitterness, and anger engendered by a positive AIDS diagnosis, the individual and his/her support network were finally able to make some decisions based on the fairly certain fatality of the disease.

Those who found themselves in the confusing and rapidly chang-ing gray zone were often nearly immobilized by the lack of definition and clear prognosis for the ARC diagnosis. Men and women with ARC daily confronted the possibility of developing AIDS; they could neither distance themselves nor come to grips with having a fatal illness. In addition, broad speculation about a carrier state threw people in the ARC category into another type of panic and fear. Perhaps they were the Typhoid Marys of AIDS; perhaps they had given the disease to friends or lovers already. The "worried well" could still distance them-selves from AIDS. If they had no symptoms they could hope and pretend that they had never been exposed, or would never cross the line from exposure to illness.

The announcement of the HTLV-III discovery only made matters worse for those in the ARC category and those who were worried but well. Many were led to believe that the identification of HTLV-III had signified the end of AIDS. Those who had not followed the AIDS story closely had a false hope that the cure was just around the corner, or that a simple test would tell them whether or not they had AIDS. The cruelly and misleadingly optimistic media coverage caused many gay men to return to behaviors they had engaged in before the appearance of AIDS, behavior which many doctors and AIDS activists believe increases the possibility of contracting AIDS. Those who were not fully cognizant of the political maneuverings surrounding the HTLV-III reporting saw Margaret Heckler's announcement as an indication that the government was finally stepping in to allocate resources more appropriately.

HTLV-III positivity created a new category on the AIDS continuum, but the test had no more value than the observation of ARC or lymphadenopathy in predicting who would progress to AIDS. Although many claimed that HTLV-III correlated highly with lymphadenopathy, it still served only as an objective marker for an uncertain diagnosis. It became a sort of reverse placebo: those with the mysterious ARC could now have a test to see if they harbored the virus which might or might not be causing their symptoms through mechanisms not well understood. Although some gay men feel they gain knowledge from the tests, many participants in medical studies experienced an unexpected panic when they found themselves to be HTLV-III positive. To compound this uncertainty, doctors diverged widely in their opinions of the significance of a positive test. Some activists and scientists discounted the test altogether, while Gallo continues to assert that positivity means presumed communicability and asserted that the existence of the virus is the most significant factor in the onset of disease.[6]

Almost immediately, influential members of the AIDS activist community came out strongly against the test and discouraged gay men from getting it. They argued that the test placed seropositive men in undue mental stress and endangered them should the test results be obtained by an employer or insurance company.[7] There was widespread fear that the HTLV-III positive list would become a hit list for rounding up gay men. In addition, there was concern that people in high risk groups would be required to submit to HTLV-III testing (a proposal which was made in West Germany), and early non-cooperation or subversion of testing seemed the best course.

The existence of an apparently simple test makes individual quarrantine or the closing of gay establishments more tempting. The discovery of HTLV-III reinforced the reality that any solution to AIDS must be as political as it is medical. AIDS is double jeopardy: it endangers life through both disease and political persecution, and increases the likelihood that the at-risk populations will be considered guilty (infected) until proven innocent (disease-free). No solution of the AIDS epidemic will be complete until those at risk are neither blamed for the disease nor forced to live in continued fear for their lives.

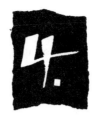

# AIDS 1985: The Atlanta Update

The International Conference on Acquired Immunodeficiency Syndrome (AIDS), held in Atlanta, Georgia in April 1985, proved to be a bleak affair for the 2,200 medical researchers and lay AIDS activists who attended. In four days of hundreds of presentations from around the world no exciting new possibilities emerged. The worst fears were confirmed: AIDS is increasing and more difficult to crack than anyone expected. But it was not only the climbing caseload figures that were distressing.

A subtle shift in the tone of discussion about preventative measures signaled increasing legal and civil rights battles for those at risk. There were differences of opinion between researchers about public health measures. Those who were ready to pull out the stops were accused of not understanding the psychology of the groups at risk. International researchers also expressed concern: they viewed the U.S. fixation on AIDS as a "gay" or "lifestyle" disease as obscuring the role of poverty, at least in third world AIDS.

The new HTLV-III/LAV test, licensed only as a blood screening device and specifically *not* as a diagnostic tool, became the battleground for these differing opinions. A minority heralded the test as a mechanism for "educating" those at risk by using mass testing as an occasion for somber contemplation of the epidemic. They argued that testing positive for the antibody should be presumed to mean infectiousness, a controversial claim not yet supported by data. One researcher reported on a study in which gay men said they wanted to take the test in order to effect changes in their sexual behavior, even though the sexual practice guidelines are the same whether one tests positive or negative, and no different from those widely publicized before the test was available.[1] The idea that gay men would choose to take a test which they admitted provided no new information testified to the mystical power this simple act could hold for panicking communities waiting for something, *anything* to emerge from medical research. Those who favored mass testing asserted people's need to know and rested firm in their belief that rational behavioral changes would result from knowledge of antibody status. They discounted legal repercussions for those tested. However, almost immediately after the conference the Armed Services issued a directive to blood collection centers to hand over the names of donors who tested positive.[2]

The politicians who were granted this captive audience had equally distressing remarks. Massachusetts' own Margaret Heckler, now Secretary of Health and Human Services, was late, as usual, and appeared to have neither written nor read her speech before its maiden voyage in the plenary session. Her use of overdrawn military metaphors embarrassed the U.S. researchers who had to sit through Heckler's mangled pronunciation of common medical terms in front of colleagues from thirty countries. Heckler said she wished "to speed the mobilization of an international war on AIDS" to end the "murderous mystery." "We have aimed our largest scientific cannon on the AIDS target, and we've had some hits." "We have succeeded: we have broken the code." Her speech writer may well have written scripts for old Reagan war films.

When Heckler reported that the HTLV-III/LAV test manufacturers had "filled the backlog of domestic orders" and that "the manufacturers have informed me that they will be able to increase production and can now turn their attention to international demands," one was reminded of the long and sordid U.S. history of pawning off unlicenseable or inappropriate medical wonders on developing nations that lack the resources to verify or implement programs designed by pharmaceutical company public relations men. Finally, she advocated an "all out war on the HTLV-III virus" (didn't she declare that last year?) to "stop the spread of AIDS before it hits the heterosexual community," a statement which offended not only gay and lesbian scientists and health activists, but also drew fire from international representatives.

Fakhry Assaad, from the World Health Organization in Geneva, took a subtle broadside at the U.S. response to AIDS: "AIDS may already have existed in developing countries five, ten, or perhaps more years. I hope solutions will be proposed and debated. I hope they will be relevant to developing nations."

Internationally, AIDS is a major health problem, complicated by the lack of knowledge about AIDS outside the massive U.S. urban gay ghettos and the lack of adequate facilities for surveillance in developing nations. WHO officials advocated implementing international use of the Centers for Disease Control's case definitions and guidelines. However, other researchers expressed concern that poverty makes AIDS difficult to identify because of the assumption of "previous health." Even in the U.S. poverty-associated disease patterns are beginning to confuse the AIDS picture. A recent study of increased tuberculosis rates in greater New York City showed that higher rates occurred in areas that were also showing increasing numbers of AIDS cases.[3] From the beginning, the secondary infections associated with AIDS have varied somewhat from one risk group to another and in different areas of the country. The tuberculosis data, and an unaccountable outbreak of AIDS in a small, very poor town in rural Florida with high levels of parasitic disease, may help to make a case for expanding the definition of AIDS.[4]

The U.S., Canada, Western Europe, and Australia show similar patterns of incidence and increase, mainly among gay/bisexual men, with the exception that the U.S. has a large and geographically clustered group of IV drug-associated AIDS cases.[5] Hemophiliac or transfusion-associated AIDS occurs only in areas with a high incidence of AIDS, or which import blood from areas with a high incidence of AIDS, such as the U.S., where blood is a major business. One wonders whether the move to "clean up" the U.S. blood supply is totally altruistic: "bad blood" may be "bad business" for this major U.S. industry.

Africa has now seen AIDS in eighteen countries, though most heavily in Zaire and the Congo. According to statistics presented by Jean Baptiste Brunet, from the World Health Organization Collaborating Center for AIDS in Paris, 50 percent of the African cases had traveled to Europe before the onset of symptoms. He strongly advocated research into migration patterns, both sexual community-related migration, as in the U.S. and Western Europe in the 1960s and 1970s, and development-related migration. The AIDS cases in Haiti and Zaire, he noted, had occurred about fifteen years after major Haitian emigration to Zaire.

The studies of Haitians, who were recently removed from the list of groups at risk, were controversial. Reports showed that *some* Haitians were at increased risk, but suggested that number of sexual partners, having emigrated to the U.S. through the Krome North detention camp, and number of non-medical injections while in Haiti were the significant risk factors.[6] It is common in Haiti and some other developing nations to receive mass innoculations of vitamins or antibiotics from minimally trained personnel at home or in the equivalent of a drugstore.

By contrast, a study of AIDS in the Dominican Republic, which shares the same island as Haiti, showed no known AIDS cases in people living solely in the D.R. In a study done at a VD clinic and a drug abuse center, persons tested showed only a 1 percent incidence of the presence of HTLV-III/LAV antibody. A small group of male homosexual prostitutes from a popular coastal resort, however, showed a 10 percent rate of the antibody to the virus. Researchers were also able to recover virus from 10 percent of a very small sample of the 15,000 to 20,000 Haitian migrant workers who come to the Dominican Republic each year to cut cane.[7]

## Out of Africa

Everyone awaited the unveiling of the African data which had attracted attention the week before the conference when a sensational (and grossly inaccurate) Knight-Ridder wire report touted proof that "household contact causes AIDS."[8] The study drew a great deal of criticism and outright hostility from scientists who have grown disgusted by inaccurate reports which they feel some colleagues do little to discourage.

The study did indeed show that those people who lived in the household of a person with AIDS more often tested positive for the HTLV-III/LAV antibody. However, the study noted, that does not mean that the person with AIDS necessarily transmitted the virus to others: "The person affected and the person who introduced the virus are not necessarily the same." As researchers from Africa and Haiti were continually to point out, due to lack of resources medical practices in developing nations do not follow the same precautions as are taken in developed countries. The study concluded that the household should be considered as a cluster of people who may have engaged in a common activity which exposed them to the virus, such as having been innoculated with the same needle.

A study of prostitutes in Rwanda (east of Zaire) showed the problem of health care surveillance in economically depressed areas,[9] a problem also found in the self-assessment of health status among poor people in the U.S. Seventy prostitutes and twenty-five of their clients recruited from a VD clinic were studied for a range of immune system problems. Although the prostitutes all reported being "well," each showed low-grade ARC-like symptoms such as fatigue, lymphadenopathy, night sweats, etc. HTLV-III/LAV antibody status in both the men and women correlated with previous VD history and number of partners. One researcher criticized the methodology of such studies, archly suggesting that, given the inadequacies of medical practice in developing nations, VD clinic patients might have contracted AIDS while being innoculated as treatment, making the risk factor *attending* a VD clinic rather than previous VD history.

Many questions were raised in response to studies claiming that prostitutes harbor AIDS and are spreading it to male customers. Certainly, various bits of data support the idea through *statistical* correlation. But the key studies cited all have major flaws, and comparison between the U.S. and Africa is fraught with differences in reporting, cultural attitudes and definitions of sexuality, and vastly different levels of medical practice. The highly reported Army study, citing numerous soldiers who denied IV drug use or homosexual contact but who claimed to have visited prostitutes in far flung places, came under attack from many researchers. No one has proposed an adequate female-to-male transmission model which might be tested. Most statistical work on gay males or female partners of male IV drug users places the person receiving semen at much greater risk. Isolated studies in some very special cases have suggested that saliva may play a role in transmission under little-understood circumstances. The very low incidence of AIDS among even "promiscuous" heterosexuals in the U.S., however, makes many researchers skeptical. There are very few cases of men getting AIDS for unaccountable reasons in the U.S.; "heterosexual" cases are far more often women who have contracted it from their male partners at risk for AIDS. Although the 50/50 gender distribution of AIDS in Africa is not understood, neither the data nor the theoretical models support blanket comparison between these and U.S. cases.

## Women and children last

The lack of attention to women with AIDS until the recent assertion that prostitutes were spreading AIDS has created a twofold problem. Some 700 women with AIDS in the U.S. are submerged in other risk categories, primarily IV drug users or sexual partners of men at risk ("other"). This has downplayed the incidence of AIDS in women and has hidden the special problems AIDS creates for women, especially in pregnancy. Thus, few women even realize that having AIDS or ARC, and perhaps even positive antibody status, may place them at higher risk for pregnancy mortality and possible transmission to fetus.

One of the least-addressed problems to date has been the appearance of some 100 cases of AIDS in children. Although the media is fond of sick baby stories, few scientists have launched major efforts to understand the parameters of AIDS in children. Not surprisingly, the majority of the pediatric cases occur in areas with greater numbers of women with AIDS—among Haitians, prostitutes, and IV drug users. Children with AIDS, ARC, and possibly HTLV-III/LAV positivity create enormous public policy problems—already experienced in Miami, New York, and New Jersey—concerning day care and schools, adoption for children whose mothers die, and combating the extreme reactions of parents who wrongly fear that their children might get AIDS through "casual contact" at school. Although studies of siblings of these children show no ill effects of "household contact," families become panic-stricken, and even children of parents imagined to be at risk for AIDS are subject to discrimination.[10]

About 70 percent of the U.S. pediatric cases are attributed to the mother's intravenous drug use, or her sexual relationship with a male with or at risk for AIDS. Seventy-five percent are black or hispanic; most of the few white cases have been attributed to transfusions.

The secondary illnesses associated with pediatric AIDS and ARC compound the problem of detection, since they are more diffuse and difficult to observe in these cases, 91 percent of whom are children under the age of three. Pneumocistis carinii pneumonia (a common agent in the environment seen dramatically in child concentration camp and war zone survivors after World War II), though consistent with the manifestations of adult AIDS, is much more difficult to diagnose in children because of the large number of childhood respiratory problems. An unusual finding was the high incidence of disseminated cytomegalo virus (CMV) as a fatal complication in children.[11] This virus has been studied in association with Kaposi's sarcoma in the long-acting, endemic KS cases in Africa, and is under investigation as a co-factor in gay men, where CMV is extremely common and in whom KS is a major manifestation of AIDS. Why so few children manifest KS, but still have high proportions of CMV, is a question of importance in the total AIDS picture.

Preliminary results of a study of sixteen mothers in Miami who had one or more children while seropositive for HTLV-III/LAV identified transmissibility of virus.[12] Eleven of these sixteen women were at risk due to male partners with or at risk for AIDS. The study found that the virus was transmissible to a fetus, but not necessarily transmitted. Some mothers who had a first seropositive infant had a second, while others delivered subsequent seronegative (normal) children. About one third of the babies were normal, one third rapidly developed AIDS, and one third developed ARC within six months of delivery. Pregnancy complications were much greater in these women.

A New Jersey study showed that four of five women who were at risk because of an IV drug-using sexual partner were and are still totally asymptomatic, but gave birth to babies with frank AIDS.[13] Women in this study showed marked increase in pregnancy mortality or complications soon after delivery.

Both the appearance of and solution to AIDS and ARC in women and their children rest on a health care system already biased against the needs of poor people of color, and especially IV drug users who fear that contact with municipal agencies may result in legal action. Some of these women may be prostitutes, whose livelihood places them at risk for AIDS but at the same time discourages them from meeting their own health care needs through traditional channels.

## HTLV-III/LAV

The amount and sophistication of the evidence linking HTLV-III/LAV to AIDS was matched only by its inability to explain why one person exposed to the virus gets AIDS while another does not. What is emerging both clinically and in the statistical data is that HTLV-III/LAV infections produce a wide range of manifestations from apparently nothing beyond an antibody response to full-blown, classic AIDS. Of course, no one really understands why one person gets the flu and another does not but the stakes are much higher with AIDS. With no treatment or cure, one faces probable death, and since the at-risk groups are already stigmatized for other reasons, mere association with the viral agent believed to cause the disease may result in discrimination. Some doctors have moved toward calling this spectrum of illness "HTLV-III disease," which makes merely testing positive for the virus a mark of "disease" rather than some constellation of identifiable symptoms. This may soften the stigma of full-blown AIDS, but only at the expense of further harming at-risk individuals by implying that anyone positive for the virus (and the at-risk groups do show higher rates of positivity) is potentially contagious. At present, data on who is infectious and when is theoretical: some researchers argue that anyone who tests positive for HTLV-III/LAV must be presumed to be infectious, while others criticize their colleagues for the hysteria this type of position creates. Most agree that the majority of people who have HTLV-III virus are at some point "shedding virus"; in other words, they can pass virus in certain body fluids under certain conditions. Exactly what those conditions are—some forms of sexual contact, but possibly saliva contact with a torn mucous membrane—are unknown. If there are significant factors such as heredity, additional current or past infections, dose factors, etc., these are not yet known.

A small but vocal minority of researchers advocated mass testing of at-risk individuals as a public health and/or educational technique. CDC official Donald Francis (though disclaiming his position as not that of the CDC) said it was inevitable that mass testing would become part of the total AIDS prevention picture. Gay men would demand to be tested because "they need to know," he asserted humans "do better in positions of knowledge." He offered charts and diagrams of which gay men could have sex with whom and which he proposed would lend order to "randomized patterns of sex" that lead to increased transmission of AIDS. But exactly what the "knowledge" of a positive or negative test was to mean in terms of real behavioral changes was unclear, and the anecdotal evidence of the many people involved in counseling gay men and IV drug users about risk reduction for AIDS pointed to dramatically different reactions of individuals once they were tested.

Gay activist Bruce Voeller also advocated mass testing as part of the educational program for gay men at risk for AIDS.[14] Based on his own experience, he claimed that gay men would change their sexual behaviors if confronted with a positive test. But activists from the various AIDS organizations questioned this logic. If the risk reduction guidelines remain the same whether you have the test or not, and even whether you test positive or not, what is gained by taking the test? James D'Eramo asked hyperbolically where the test results of gay men would be branded, and countered Francis's assertion about the efficacy of knowledge with the statement that "in knowledge, there is not necessarily wisdom."

Dr. Ken Mayer, a researcher and clinician at Boston's Fenway Community Health Center, and Professor of Medicine at Brown University, described the position of those making risk reduction guidelines and other policies as "between a rock and a hard place." He said that too many questions remained to base all one's programs on the test. These questions included: lack of understanding of the basic biology of the retrovirus; differences in susceptibility depending on the route of entry; and the very present but unknown co-factors. He was guarded about the proposal to institute a massive testing effort: "A blanket program which is perceived as an unfair infringement may alienate the people we're trying to work with." He pointed to a credibility problem in the health education efforts. Rather than a massive, simplistic testing program, he advocated greater efforts toward more extensive education. "We don't give people enough credit. We need to make hierarchies of risk, but explain the data and that it is still controversial. The epidemic is continually evolving, so we must make relative guidelines—they may be good for the present, but may change."

Issues of confidentiality loomed large in the discussion of the merits of the test. Activists cited cases of discrimination that had already occurred before the test was even put into public use. But lest these community activists feel paranoid, none other than Edward Brandt, Assistant Director of Health and Human Services echoed their concerns. Though Brandt denies it, many AIDS activists viewed his resignation from that position as political victimization. He had pushed the administration to spend more money on AIDS, and after a several-month delay was told by Margaret Heckler to shift funds around. Although he was never openly critical of the Reagan administration, Brandt's views were always out of step with the right-wing attitude of shifting health care costs and concerns to state and local levels. Since his resignation in late 1984, Brandt has openly admitted that the administration had proposed mass quarantine (which he opposed), had never understood the complexity of the problem, and had allowed social prejudices to cloud the policy issues.[15] His conclusion from this experience was well received by those attending the Atlanta conference:

> I think it is necessary for the scientific community to take the time to study the full biological and social implications of this disease in order to learn for the future. That is difficult to undertake in the current political climate. But we should be concerned with discovering truth rather than disclosing error.

He expressed concern about the difficulty of studying a disease whose two hardest hit groups face great legal and social repercussions because "of the strong views of people in this society." He stated that confidentiality was of equal relevance for those uncovering medical aspects of the disease because "numerous groups would bring pressure to reveal names." Echoing the concerns of many of the local groups over mass testing plans and sensationalized media reports, Brandt said, "I don't believe that scare tactics accomplish information exchange. Informational and educational programs are important. People affected must be cared for and not subjected to the discrimination that we have

already seen." He reaffirmed his conviction while still part of the
Reagan administration, a view which was voiced by almost everyone
else at the conference: "We need a national funding effort. Throwing
money at a problem doesn't help, but starving it doesn't help either."

It was the summary data on the seroprevalence of HTLV-III/LAV
in at-risk populations which engendered the greatest sense of despair at
this conference. Studies of gay men in New York City, Washington,
D.C., Denmark, San Francisco, and smaller cities like Boston and
Pittsburgh, as well as studies of hemophiliacs using Factor VIII (a
compound made from many blood donors) and of IV drug users in New
York and New Jersey, confirmed what has long been feared. Retrospective studies of stored serum (from previous studies of other diseases)
show HTLV-III/LAV with a low prevalence but increasingly prevalent
as long as two years before the first case of AIDS in an area. The
seroprevalence curves reach as high as 30 or 40 percent in some cases
before the first AIDS cases appear. The curve depicting AIDS cases then
follows in direct proportion to the prevalence of HTLV-III/LAV about
two years before.[16] The problem with the long incubation periods
found in AIDS is that most communities do not respond until there is a
critical mass of AIDS cases, and by then the seroprevalence is already
quite high. Doomsday interpretations of this data assume that 10 to 40
percent of these people will eventually get AIDS or fatal cases of ARC,
but without data on co-factors (especially in different populations)
such figures seem overly fatalistic. Risk reduction education efforts
have shown good results in the smaller, and hence later-affected cities,
which many hope will slow or halt increases in overall seroprevalence
in those areas. Still, the uncertainty about co-factors, the rate of
unchecked increase in seroprevalence, and the actual number of AIDS
cases predictable from current seroprevalence rates pose a dire picture.

## Virology

The lack of treatment and cure for AIDS is due to the retroviral nature of
the HTLV-III/LAV. Retroviruses have only been under study for about
a dozen years, and their basic biology is still not well understood.

Viruses of any variety are not quite living organisms, like bacteria
or parasites. They are pieces of protein encased in an envelope, a simple
biological building block which needs a home in order to pursue its life
process. Most viruses are chunks of DNA—the basic genetic material in
all cells. Retroviruses are RNA, a component which works with DNA
in cell-division processes. In retroviruses, replication happens back-
wards: instead of going from DNA through RNA to produce daughter

DNA, the retrovirus begins with RNA and then an enzyme called reverse transcriptase acts on the RNA to produce DNA. Once inside a host cell, the HTLV-III/LAV, for example, produces this DNA, which penetrates the core of the host cell and attempts to integrate itself at certain points in the host cell's DNA. If successful, the retrovirus's transcribed RNA is ever after part of that cell's genetic code. It is not clear whether this integration in and of itself is sufficient to disrupt the cell's processes, or whether additional factors inside the host cell, or outside in the plasma, are necessary for the severe immune dysfunction seen in classic AIDS. The T-4 cell, which is the favorite home of HTLV-III/LAV, sits at a critical place in total immune function; if it is not operating properly, a whole series of malfunctions occurs. However, it is not clear whether this immuno deficiency represents a single chain of events; a progressive but interactive process with other genetic factors or other viruses; or even repeat assaults of HTLV-III/LAV. Virologists and immunologists do not agree among themselves about how HTLV-III/LAV works, alone or in concert, to effect the total, systemic breakdown witnessed in AIDS.

One method of determining how HTLV-III/LAV works is to try a range of therapies acting at different points in the virus/host interaction. Immuno modulators such as the interferons, as well as drugs like suramin, have been tried on patients with AIDS and even the earlier stages of ARC. To date, no single therapy seems capable of halting or reversing the effects of immune suppression in these patients. However, several of the therapies seem to address part of the complex of problems seen at the cellular level. Researchers are beginning to pursue combination therapies that address several aspects of immune breakdown at once. Dr. Martin Hirsch, a researcher at Massachusetts General Hospital, recommended rapid development of combination therapies.[17] He also advocated retesting some drugs on less immune-compromised patients. The confusing nature of retroviruses might mean that treatment could be very long, he said, "even lifetime." In Hirsch's, as well as most other researchers' estimation, there is a "long way to go before AIDS is preventable or treatable."

The conference participants seemed to have grown weary of AIDS, and not solely because of the sadness and frustration of dealing with the patients of such a devastating disease. (Indeed, plenty of researchers have never actually seen a person with AIDS.) The novelty of a fascinating new disease to conquer is wearing thin: in the uneasy marriage of (mostly) straight researchers and mostly gay or drug-user guinea pigs, the honeymoon is over. Everyone needs someone to blame for the disease and for the failure to find significant treatments, methods of prevention, or cures. But even while the computers, statisticians, and brilliant and creative minds of the worldwide scientific community had no good news, and little that was even novel, those working with the at-risk groups left with a sense of grim determination: they would work harder to design better, more refined tools for educating and support-ing their constituents.

# SECTION TWO
# The Body Besieged

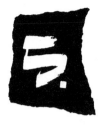

# Germphobia

The idea that AIDS is transmitted by a germ, a tiny microscopic agent, complicates both social and political reactions to the illness. Germphobia is triggered whether or not there is an "AIDS germ," producing irrational, visceral responses when least expected. Germphobic panic appears despite rational understanding of the etiology and communicability of AIDS. Arguing with unknowledgeable friends or colleagues that AIDS can't be passed through casual contact coexists with the gripping, unexpected jolt of fear at the affectionate goodbye kiss of a gay male friend.

Contemporary concern with germs is ironic: the public is subject to fewer deadly germs than recent ancestors, U.S. medical practice can more readily identify and cope with those that remain. Yet the fear of germs—codified during the Lysol and plastic-packaged 1950s—verges on a mass psychosis. Germs are bad guys: foreign, unnegotiable, dangerous. Despite popular films and articles which describe a multitude of microbes that live happily and even helpfully within the body, the middle-class melting pot mentality views the body as pristine, clean, uninvaded, untouched until germs tread on this wholesome purity. U.S. culture views the human body, like the "virgin" land of the new world, as the site of a passionate battle between good and evil, order and chaos, health and disease. If U.S. manifest destiny is exhibited by the number of savages conquered, the number of wildernesses domesticated, then the conquest of the body is measured by physical prowess and freedom from an ever-changing definition of disease.

## Plagues and science

Despite contemporary attacks on medicine as big business, and even some doubt about the efficacy of this scientific endeavor, most U.S. citizens reserve special awe for the *idea* of modern medicine. Doctors are greeted with suspicion and "alternative" forms of medicine have become increasingly popular, but when it comes right down to the life-threatening or calamitous, most people opt for the boys in white. Modern Western medicine has achieved its stranglehold on the delivery of a wide range of bodily care only in this century, and in the last three decades the organization of medical care has reached the proportions of an industrial empire. The meaning and nature of medical knowledge have changed, and with them, the social and psychological relationship between the individuals who hold title to that knowledge and the clients who benefit from trade secrets.

In absolute terms, knowledge of the human body and the disturbances that affect it has increased since the advent of scientific medicine. The type of knowledge gained, and its relationship to actual human health needs, however, are subjects of much debate.[1] Medicine is popularly believed to solve the problems of sickness by finding cures for whichever diseases ravage the human population at any given point. Actually, many "plague" diseases—characterized by sudden or new appearance and rampant form—limit themselves *before* doctors discover a "cure."[2]

Beliefs about how disease operates have changed radically with modern medicine, yet diseases simple and complex continue to elude medical science. Cancer remains a mystery, and influenza—though less fatal than fifty years ago—still strikes cyclically. In fact, while flu vaccines are continually improved, rapidly mutating new influenza strains are often a step ahead in their quest to find a home in the human body.[3] The Centers for Disease Control scientists use their information about flu patterns to predict which strains will appear next. Sometimes they guess correctly, but when wrong the flu vaccine has been as dangerous to at-risk populations (the very young, very old, and chronically ill) as the viruses themselves.

The contemporary U.S. experience of relative freedom from disease heightens the belief that doctors can stop epidemics. Often researchers can do little more than study the disease's natural history and prevent recurrence or spread outside the initial target population. Epidemiology is the branch of medicine that studies and copes with epidemics. Although this science has a century-long history and well-developed methods, the general public only dimly understands the nature of the epidemics it studies.

Epidemics are not a contest between doctors and germs, fought on the turf of the human body. Epidemics have their own ecological mechanisms, and depend on a wide range of factors that have as much to do with social and demographic specifics as the particular qualities of the infectious agent. McNeil suggests that it is useful to view epidemics from the germs' point of view. Human beings exist in a wide network of parasitic and symbiotic relationships with germs. Micro-organisms have an interest in their host's well-being, since the host provides a home. From the standpoint of these micro-organisms, producing illness is functional, but killing the host is not. Virulent micro-organisms can only survive if there is an infinite number of possible hosts linked by one or more transmission routes. Epidemics are self-limiting and cyclical as a function of host mass and resistance, ease of transmission, mutability of host and microbe, and viability of microbe outside the human body. The major epidemics of the past occurred in regular cycles. Cholera would appear, reach epidemic proportions, then lose ground through depletion of hosts. With bacterial infections, the first epidemics are often the most virulent. Exposed survivors produce antibody so that a second attack produces fewer casualties. Some of the epidemic diseases of the past became more frequent but less devastating as the human hosts and microbial agent reached a balance.

Vaccination is a crude imitation of this natural negotiation process between agent and hosts. A vaccine provides a controlled exposure to a small enough dose to trigger an antibody response without also producing full-blown symptoms. Vaccines provide one method of preventing recurrence of an epidemic disease. But the vaccine merely deprives the agent of a suitable home; it does not end the disease itself. Although the major classic epidemic diseases are under control in the U.S., there are still occasional outbreaks in isolated circumstances where the microbes have lain dormant awaiting the proper human host environment.[4]

Curing infected individuals is a more time-consuming operation, which does not prevent the reintroduction of the agent into a population. Many contemporary diseases are easily eliminated in the individual with safe drugs. The relative value of drugs versus vaccines as methods of stemming the tide of disease depends on the efficacy and safety of the intervention and the severity of the disease.

The final method for containing disease is to break the chain of transmission. Epidemiologists frequently refer to John Snow, founder of their discipline, who—against the scientific wisdom of his day—deduced that a sudden epidemic was centered around a certain water pump in London.[5] When he removed the handle of the pump, so the folklore goes, the epidemic was halted. It was fifty years before other scientists accepted germ theory and the transmission pattern alleged in Snow's study. Snow was ridiculed and died in obscurity. Despite still unclear transmission routes in AIDS, more than one scientist has suggested "removing the pump handle" from the gay community.

## The domestication of germs

Until the 1700s, Western science was concerned with essence, and with elaborating the laws governing the *regularity* of events. The Aristotelian world view circumscribed the very objects of inquiry: in medicine, the body was viewed as a whole, organic process that mediated life and death. Although pre-germ theories of health varied in some details, early Western medicine basically viewed disease as an imbalance of life-sustaining elements, an imbalance that could be discovered only through the patient's subjective description of pains and moods. These early systems lacked any but the crudest medical technology, and the production of medical knowledge consisted of generalizing about and predicting the course of bodily changes that would result in illness or health.

Pre-rational holism integrated functions and symptoms now considered discrete.[6] Disease and symptoms were viewed as identical: symptoms *were* the disease, not indications of an underlying problem. The conflation of disease and symptoms permitted some diseases to make a patient seem exotic, gifted, spiritual, and not *disordered*.[7] A typically absurd conclusion of the organic theories which reverberates today was the claim that aggressive acting-out of upper-class nineteenth-century women reflected a disorder of the uterus—hence the name "hysteria."[8] These women's behavior could be categorized as physical illness, a product of defective breeding equipment—and thereby discouraged and controlled, since the ability to breed was one of the values placed on these women.

Under pre-scientific medicine, intervention in disease meant restoring the disturbed balance. But since disease was not considered to be located or fixed in any one part of the body (constituting instead a referred system superimposed on the body), treatment was often ineffective or worse. The extreme concern for balance in the whole person eclipsed attention to problems in subsystems and limited the usefulness of early medical knowledge. The unified theory of the corporeal is a compelling notion which resonates through the generations of scientific biology: enhancing one part of the system, even if capriciously defined, in order to restore balance to the whole would later find expression in the modern holistic approach, and even in the science of immunology. Medical mysticism echoes the critical concern for beefing up the immune system, which like the humors of the homeo-path is omnipresent, not in a *particular* location—creating a potential for retaliatory action if disease arises, and standing as an invisible militia prepared for deployment in search of anomaly.

If pre-germ theory doctors had special knowledge based on an understanding of the body's supposed balancing act and the proper interpretation of a patient's recitation of complaints, post-germ theory doctors had an even more powerful claim to knowledge. Evolving technologies gave doctors real and apparent ability to see what the patient could not. The introduction of the anatomical method in the 1700s began a shift toward "the gaze."[9]

The emergence of epidemiology in the mid-1800s highlighted the importance of understanding the disease's course through a *popula-tion*, not just in an individual. Instead of looking only for what was out of balance in the individual, the new method sought to uncover factors which differentiated the sick from the well. Disease became objective and observable through case comparison, rather than being intensely subjective, requiring extensive input and description from the sick person. A self-presentation which might be considered suspiciously hypochondriacal today was the primary data solicited by the pre-germ theory doctor. The doctor's power as a gatekeeper to the benefits of sickness and health has increased with the modern objective methods which may declare a health status at odds with the patient's impression.

A new philosophy was necessary for medicine to shift from the whole to parts. Descarte's mechanistic view of the body not only split the mental and physical, but ultimately laid the foundation for viewing the body as a separate system of interrelated but autonomous pro-cesses.[10] But the mechanistic view could not suddenly and totally replace the longstanding notion of a balance of primal elements, nor was the old idea of holism completely without virtue. Even though the mechanistic view of the body and of disease permitted analysis of individual diseases and created the possibility of vaccines, antibiotics, and anesthesia, the medical technology to develop them was not yet available. The shift in world view went hand in hand with increasingly available technologies: as medical imagination hypothesized more dis-crete functions, medical technologists sought innovations that would permit literal seeing.

Industrialization allowed for more rapid production of these new ways of observing people at the same time that humans were consoli-dated in one place to be observed in urban clinics and hospitals. The intensification of social anxiety of the new class structure facilitated the creation of a *class* of patients, as well as the means for reinforcing their status through technologies aimed at comparison of cases rather than comprehension of individual problems.

The new medical science inherited from its predecessor the search for essence, redefined as basic measurable ("seeable") building blocks. As each medical fantasy found its technological reality (or was debunked as nonsense if no technology could be found to anchor its existence), a new fantasy was created. Each smallest part seemed to yield up yet smaller components. New technologies were sought to resolve the inconsistency or problems revealed by the previous breakthrough: medical scientists theorized increasingly complex formulas of bodily operation. The human body was ever more fragmented, as scientists sought to view smaller parts out of their context. Indeed, the rapidly decreasing size of the object of inquiry made the human body as a whole seem crude and irrelevant. The mysterious and organic became the visible and demonstrable. During the 1800s the theoretical, practical, and technological conditions were laid for isolating causal factors from incidental, and by the mid-1900s bacterial and amoebic disorders would be fairly easy to conquer.

## Secular disease

Before the popularization of germ theory at the turn of this century, disease, particularly in epidemic form, was thought to be caused by God. This method of sorting out the good from the bad was particularly insidious, since disease could hide inside the contours of the human body, could locate and punish hidden sins and infractions. The idea that disease was an act of God was particularly malleable and interpreted by clergy to suit their needs as arbitrators of morality and interpreters of group differences. This old notion of disease as signifier of sin expanded the power of the church to enforce social codes.

Pre-germ theory doctors were little better than handmaidens to the rich, one type of healer among many. The middle-class healers, who would evolve into the prestigious medical doctors of today, occupied a social status between the proletariat and the aristocracy. They depended entirely on the rich for their income, either directly, through care of wealthy clients, or indirectly through subsidies to clean up the poor.[11] Not surprisingly, illness in the rich carried fewer hints of moral causation, and might be attributed to living in a world polluted by immoral people and the poor (not the more ubiquitous "polluted" environment often seen as causal today). Disease in the rich, especially tuberculosis, could even be a sign of purity or special sensitivity.

Disease in the working classes experienced a script rewrite commensurate with the new values of an industrialized world. God no longer caused disease directly, but "his" weaker human creations met with increased hazards. The poor were not viewed as a class of disadvantaged people; rather, poverty was seen as the punishment for racial, or cultural difference. Sloth, vice, and overcrowding were increasingly viewed as the *causes*, not the results of poverty. Disease was verification that the poor, through the constellation of factors that marked their poverty, were indeed inferior and immoral.[12]

The dirt of poverty replaced the disorder of sin: poverty and sin were equivalent, and disease stood as the sign and punishment for either. By a curious twist of logic, disease in the poor retained the power of moral stigma—the slothful poor attracted their diseases—while the exact same disease in the wealthy was caused by microbes unleashed by *others*. The shifting gender and class relations in the rapidly industrializing U.S. left much room for interpretation of who got sick and why. Only venereal disease remained classified by the part of the body attacked and stood as proof of contact with immorality and disorder, regardless of class or gender.

The evolution of a "working class" which came in close contact with upper classes through increased urbanization and massive industrial workplaces forced the middle-class doctor onto the working class, which had previously employed a variety of traditional healers.[13] At the turn of the century, as germ theory captured the imagination of the West, industrialization forced other changes in concepts and delivery of health care. In an age fascinated by rationalism, doctors, with their modicum of schooling, appeared scientific and easily gained presumptive power in the struggles over legitimacy that ultimately consolidated middle-class doctors into a profession.

Classes had long received different types and qualities of health care, but the consolidation of medical doctors as the health professionals for all classes affected patterns of medical intervention, in spite of the new promise of eliminating many diseases. Disease justified the existing organization of sexual and social mores between and within classes, races, and genders. The idea that natural group differences were reflected in disease patterns permitted non-intervention in certain diseases or classes. If a plague hit an unpopular class, far be it from doctors to interfere in God's—or nature's—plan. Doctors might confine the disease so that it did not spread outside its perceived appropriate class. Since cures were rare, death rationalized the hypothesis that illness was a mark of moral weakness rather than casting doubt on the efficacy of medical providers and their new-found science. Doctors' monopoly on the definition of disease and cures permits this notion to persist today; only recently has the failure to cure cancer, for example, called into question the system of scientific medicine. Cancer is popularly viewed as the result of overindulgence or emotional repression that is compounded more rapidly than the technology of cures—a contradictory view that blames the individual rather than the branch of science which has not helped humans keep pace with technology.

Likewise, AIDS and the apparent recent proliferation of homosexuality are viewed as surpassing technology's ability to adjust the wages of unnatural sex. Some people are quite happy to blame the liberal society that is imagined to have permitted homosexuality to flourish, as well as homosexuals themselves, for "causing" AIDS. AIDS, and to a lesser extent cancer, show in relief the persistence of moralized ideas about disease and the stigmatizing mechanisms they trigger. Homosexuals in the 1980s have inherited the moral paradigm of disease that in earlier decades determined the health care patterns for the black and poor.

Disease among the poor in the 1980s retains its moral overtones, as Reagan slashes the social welfare programs designed to promote health through improved nutrition, housing, and health care subsidies. Third world and a few U.S. AIDS researchers have proposed strong connections between poverty and at least AIDS secondary infections, and possibly transmission patterns.

It is the mysterious link to homosexuality, drug use, blood, and Caribbean nationals that has captured the public eye, not pre-existing patterns of medical neglect. AIDS has provided an opportunity for the right wing to focus on a sensational media event while dismantling the very community-oriented health programs that would provide sensitive care for a variety of different needs. The negative attention to AIDS that heightens moral panic rather than developing concrete policy and research solutions provides a smoke screen and a rationale for greater regulation of "public health"—especially sex—through the suppression of difference. The message is that *difference* causes diseases which have the power to leap social barriers. Individuals must conform to rigid, traditional standards in order to protect the health of the whole society.

## Public health/sexual disorder

Secularized medicine did not radically shift the answer to whose health needs were to be met, but it did describe illness and who got sick in a new way. The profound cultural fear of difference and death, rooted deep in the European experience and magnified in the U.S., was resymbolized and articulated in the field of public health. This unique community effort at social cleansing operated under the guise of scientific medicine to control those identified as deficient, immoral, or downtrodden in order to prevent the spread of their diseases (physical and spiritual) to the community at large.

Venereal germs became a special category of disease agents which were viewed as willfully contracted. If VD could no longer be considered a manifestation of moral corruption because its microbial cause was visible, then it could become an even worse disorder because its route of transmission was an act chosen in violation of social mores and religious law. Of all the diseases which served simultaneously as symptoms of evil and as punishment in themselves, VD retained both qualities in U.S. culture. At a time when Anglo-American society was intensely concerned with sexual order, sexual disease served as a powerful code.

The feminist and social purity movement activists' attack on VD stimulated the invention of the category of sexual disease. Although for dissimilar reasons, each group was concerned with protecting morally pure (middle-class) women who might contract VD from their men. Men were believed to be morally inferior and were held to less stringent sexual standards (called "the double standard").[14] These men might transport lower-class germs via prostitutes, thereby polluting the middle class with innocent transmissions. Feminists were concerned about the plight of prostitutes, but not out of fear of the effects VD had on them (Victorians often thought that diseases, especially VD, did not harm lower-class people, who supposedly had a more robust constitution—one reason why health-protective labor laws were not always of great concern). Rather, they viewed attacking VD as a method of rounding up prostitutes and reforming them on the bourgeois model. A working-class prostitute was damned by two types of social disorder: sex and class. Venereal disease was an externality of the social vice of prostitution: VD was not just a disease but a symptom of moral disorder in the lower classes, and a sign of immoral contact in the middle classes.[15]

From the beginning, the notion of public health was classist and anti-sex, even though it often appeared as a socially progressive force during the Victorian era. The increased awareness of germs in relation to venereal disease made it acceptable to discuss sex in the guise of science.[16] Germs, population control, and the slippage toward locating sin in mental disorders subjected sexuality to the impulse to categorize that was so prevalent in the turn of the century U.S.

Sexuality moved from the binary system of legal versus illegal to the shaded grays of natural versus unnatural. Before the emergence of sexology, most discussion of sex centered on what was and was not permissible within marriage—and completely proscribed anything outside. After sexology, discussion of "normal" sex was less interesting than the massive project of categorizing and differentiating the abnormal. The imposition of rationalism on carnal knowledge held mixed promise for the sexual libertines. On one hand, sexual differences became identified and seemed to proliferate in urban areas where masses of people could read or hear for the first time names for their unspoken sexual inclinations. On the other hand, the idea of ranked sexual categories, arriving concurrently with social purity movements calling for increased self-control by men, was imbued with the presumption that normal or natural sex was conducted inside the heterosexual marriage.

Though sometimes socially progressive, sexologists failed to challenge the biological basis of gender and the over-determination of gender in sexuality, a topic explored in great detail in Chapter 8. They argued for legal acceptance and tolerance for some "deviance" and "perversion," but most promoted hormonal theories of homosexuality. The late Victorian scientists had infinite faith in their ability to discover causes, and believed it would be only a matter of time before the tiny particles governing sexuality were isolated. The possibility of hypothetical tiny particles potentially visible or at least measurable through new technologies and future tests trapped a generation or more of homosexuals in a battle with biological reductionism.[17]

The notion that social experience might dwarf any biological component was soon dismissed, unless it was dredged up in horror stories of perverts recruiting others. But even in this case the recruit was not considered a true deviant, only a weak or tainted person by virtue of "contagious contact." [18] Such "victims" were seen as innocent in their perversion, much as others were innocent in their contraction of venereal disease. Creating this exempt category brought the tautology of sexual perversion full circle: an evaluation of the individual based on capricious criteria administered by medical scientists determined the status as a deviant. The study of sexuality—awaiting its germ to be made visible—inherited the pre-germ theory function of disease as an ordering mechanism. Germ theory made disease an external assault; sexual deviation became the disorder hidden within. Disease had found its objective tests; sexuality awaited its measures as a proper scientific object.

The persistently invisible "sex germ" would find a more satisfactory cultural niche in the idea of drives or desire, a further banishment *inward* to the mind or emotions. Sex retains all of the pre-germ theory notions about disease as a manifestation of moral disorder, and no amount of rational science can rescue it. As a hidden, internal disorder with an untestable cause, the possibility of discovering oneself a pervert places post-Victorians in a perpetual state of terror: the symptoms of disorder may at any time manifest themselves. Heterosexuals become obsessed with their own normalcy, even as the perverts become more overwrought about their differences. Abnormal sex placed the individual in the state of disorderliness and required some social ritual (institutionalization, therapy, marriage) to make him or her normal. Once returned to order, she or he must continually be scrutinized for relapse by an elaborate and ongoing system of sexual surveillance. The Catholic confessional became the first site and archetypal form for a confessional sexuality that psychology and all manner of "Dear Abby" and self-help groups would eventually seek to organize.[19]

## Democracy and the frontier of disease

Throughout the nineteenth-century U.S. the democratic notion of common sense and self-care vied with the demands (real and perceived) of the emerging medical profession. The application of Western medicine in the U.S. varied across immigrant cultures, and differences in practice became geographically isolated until communication lines improved in the twentieth century. Even today, "local practice" governs the legal aspects of malpractice.

Medical theory and practice in the U.S. shifted rapidly because new settlers were cut off from the European medical establishment, rendering U.S. medicine more competitive, innovative, and often unsound. Unsuccessful applicants to the medical hierarchy in Europe often moved to the U.S. bringing with them a hostility toward clinical medicine which made them simultaneously more open to democratic ideas about medicine and more protective of their emerging status.[20]

In the U.S., the forces of religious pluralism and democracy conspired to set the secular and religious magic that empowered healers and clergy in competition with a naturalistic approach to healing. The mystical and deterministic notions of disease held by Puritans and other religious separatists conflicted with the necessity of explorers and frontierspeople who had no choice but to view disease as a natural process in which they could intervene.

Medical science was based on a rationalist framework that held disease to be comprehensible. The common-sense approach of the Methodist movement in nineteenth-century England and the U.S. took this tenet of science literally, creating a series of democratic medicine movements aimed at folk cures and simple, ostensibly scientific instructional pamphlets that the average person could follow.[21] Even through the present, for all the sophisticated technological trappings of health care, there continually emerge health self-help movements to counterbalance increases in professional authority. Although almost none claim to provide a cure, the some dozen AIDS books published at the beginning of the health crisis all purport to explain the simple facts of a complex disease for the layperson. Such books provide important information, but they rarely push the reader to directly challenge the medical profession's authority and merely serve to translate the unnecessarily complicated information. Medical self-help movements criticize but also reinforce the power of medical authority by explaining without offering comprehensive solutions for reversing the trend toward increased professionalization.

The break from the European intellectual and scientific establishment allowed for the development of a new medical authority compatible with the U.S. notion that science and medicine were fundamentally understandable by the average person. Practical demands for health care made a medical career at least theoretically accessible to anyone from nearly any segment of society. Medical credentialling in the U.S. shifted away from the European system of patronage to an apparently more democratic system. A wide array of medical institutions competed for students until the early twentieth century, when medical schools were required to offer standard curricula and students were required to pass standardized licensing tests.[22]

The rationalist, free-enterprise ethos of the industrial U.S. viewed scientific products as commodities in an open market. In turn, doctors competed for patients claiming superiority based on greater scientism or more democratic application as often as demonstrated ability to heal. With the twentieth-century application of rigorous, case-controlled research the right to decide what form of medicine was most effective shifted from the consumer to the research clinician.

The competition between democratic notions of medicine and the emerging medical empire occurred on many fronts, but germ theory, and the ability to lay claim to the technologies that support it, ultimately tipped medicine into doctors' hands. The idea of democratic medicine would continually re-emerge as classes of people sought equal access to medical care or to medical credentialling, and as patients demanded greater participation in the process of deciding their medical treatment.

## Medical research: the empire strikes back

Doctors today are helpful to their grateful patients in ways large and awesome, like successful heart transplants (subsidized by insurance), and small and mundane, like prescribing antibiotics for minor infections that cause discomfort. But the *system* a patient confronts today, although it claims and even appears to be knowledgeable and sympathetic, is quite irrational and unevenly developed. Adequate patient care is directly determined by ability to pay with money or insurance. Research money goes to cure dramatic middle-class illness, while proven health maintenance programs are cut rather than improved and expanded. Cancer research is a multimillion-dollar industry in its own right, while birth control and venereal disease remedies have developed slowly and are generally still risky to the user. Cures are favored over preventive medicine in both research and practice. Treatment is more profitable than prevention, and leaves the victims of illness more vulnerable to social control than they would be as unwitting potential victims.

Anyone forced to go to a city hospital or who gets an unusual illness quickly discovers that patient care and research/teaching are symbiotically related—with research needs threatening to edge out patient comfort, and teaching dehumanizing the care process. Research, of course, may benefit patients as a part of the protocol and may also produce results which benefit everyone. But despite clinicians' sincere intentions, patients end up feeling like guinea pigs whose individual concerns are overlooked in a project that seeks to summarize data about classes of people or illness.

Research—however sincere and brilliant its practitioners—has gained eminence as the premiere medical endeavor because it perpetuates the power vested in modern medicine and is lucrative to the industry as a whole. The medical empire has a complete structure of monetary redistribution—a whole economy—that consolidates capital within the research hospitals and interfaces with an insurance system that pools the tiny medical investments of individuals who buy insurance into a vast reservoir of prepaid medical care, available for reinvestment in other industries.[23] The available purchasing power within the empire creates a giant lottery that makes liquid resources accessible to a wide variety of projects. Only with the cost containment efforts of the 1970s did the empire flex its financial muscle in a way that was obviously to the disadvantage of many patients: the cuts were reflected in lower stocks of vital supplies, decreased patient amenities, and less advantageous labor contracts.[24]

To make matters worse, the companies which supply the machines, drugs, and rubber gloves to doctors and researchers are interlocked and diversified into cosmetics, soap, automobile tires—virtually any cost-efficient line of production that employs the same research information or manufacturing techniques. The ability to use pure research discoveries about materials and processes in multiple real production situations spreads the cost and risk of research and development over several potential market sectors. If the new rubber surgical glove is superseded, the patented process may be applied to the manufacture of bicycle tires, a conglomerate's secondary line. Knowledge is further consolidated in the maze of patents, and capital remains in the nearly hermetic economy of the empire. Computers for hospitals and research firms have found an increasing market in the past fifteen years (in part because the requirements for coordinating the information of an increasingly complex and irrationally organized system are enormous), and biosynthesizing technologies promise new possibilities for enhancing the status and wealth of medicine as a whole.[25]

The drug companies (which often have or are the secondary line of a durable goods producer) are intimately interconnected with research and clinical medicine. The first capital for research in the nineteenth-century U.S. came from the infant pharmaceutical companies who, by the turn of the century, became subject to greater regulation. Pharmacological research by clinicians was directly related to the struggle to control all medical practice: doctors viewed pharmacologists as a threat since they could prescribe drugs without a doctor's orders. Doctors gained control over drug prescription by agreeing to a direct conduit to drug companies. It became illegal for manufacturers to put recognizable common names or usage instructions on prescription drugs. In return, lawsuits and the growing legitimacy of medical doctors curtailed the manufacture and advertisement of "patent" medicines, which competed with scientific drug companies. Doctors and the emerging prescription drug industry both gained control of their domains by eliminating competing folk remedies and demoting the drug-sale middleman, the pharmacologist.[26]

Researchers and pharmaceutical companies are still in bed together: researchers are able to cut costs on projects by obtaining directly from the producer free drugs for trial use. In addition, formal drug research in a controlled clinical setting is required before most drugs are permitted on the market, reinforcing the relationship between clinicians and the drug companies. At least some of this research, most of it protected from the public eye by trade secrets laws, occurs in prisons or in populations with limited free choice due to economic or physical factors. But even this system of testing can be and often is circumvented. Once a drug is on the market for an approved ("labeled") use, a doctor is at liberty to prescribe it for additional unapproved ("unlabeled") uses. The unconscionable amount of money spent on trade journal advertising by drug companies and on personal visits from sales representatives further promotes a drug's use. Although a doctor is liable for any harm caused by an "unorthodox" use, numerous drugs have well-known and documented unlabeled uses which no one could possibly win a malpractice suit against. In fact, both the FDA (ostensibly for information-gathering reasons) and drug companies (because it creates additional markets for existing products) actually encourage thoughtful unlabeled usages. Drug companies will supply free drugs to doctors who embark on various well-designed and not-so-well designed studies, and the FDA issues policy statements such as this one:

> New uses for drugs already on the market are often first discovered through serendipitous observations and therapeutic innovations, subsequently confirmed by well-planned and executed clinical investigations.[27]

They don't mention that unlabeled uses also cause products to be removed from *any* use, and can cause great harm. Nor do they mention that drugs may continue to be employed in unlabeled use in the absence of well-planned investigations.

These "experiments"—often uncontrolled—are first anecdotally reported in medical journals, in order to garner funds for additional study. Other doctors, and in the case of Depo-Provera courts of law, begin interpreting the still undocumented use as a permitted use. The publication of these uncontrolled observations of a very few cases can lead to much more widespread use for unlabeled purposes, and these unlabeled uses become accepted medical practice without the drug ever going through the proper channels of FDA approval.

Johns Hopkins Medical School researchers have been doing "preliminary" studies on the use of Depo-Provera (the widely protested birth control injection now used only in the third world on "sex offenders" for almost two decades, despite requests from their own Institutional Review Board that they document their results in a properly designed, controlled study.[28] The incomplete and unsubstantiated Depo studies have been adopted as fact by several courts who have required Depo maintenance programs for "sex offenders" as a condition of parole. Depo, which has harmful side-effects like cancer as well as uncomfortable side-effects like weight gain, headaches, listlessness, and nausea, has through this process become acceptable for this unlabeled use, in spite of the lack of a controlled study and criticism by lawyers and other medical researchers.

Not surprisingly, in this irrational and profit-motivated medical empire, the problems of drug research can cut both ways: drugs that seem to have benefits may not be released for political reasons. Gay men with AIDS who were accepted for drug trials in a 1983 interferon program literally "died waiting" while Ronald Reagan gained international points by sending one million dollars' worth of the drug to cure the Austrian Leipziger horses of herpes infection.[29] In the case of toxic shock syndrome, the rigors of medical "proof" were so stringently applied by the scientists hired by Procter and Gamble, whose Super Rely tampon seemed to correlate highly with the 1980-81 deaths and illnesses, that plaintiffs had to embark on difficult legal maneuvers just to get the information proving their case released.[30]

# Law and Medicine

Legal authority in the U.S. emerged concurrently with the consolidation of medical authority. Although the history of the legal profession is markedly different from that of the medical profession, they are interrelated in some important ways. The last few decades have seen the emergence of three new areas of law: medical ethics, medical malpractice, and the civil rights of the disabled (defined by medical and psychological standards). From one perspective, it seems that as medicine grew in stature to protect humans from germs, law expanded in scope to protect people from science and doctors. Medicine and law have had a paradoxical relationship in these last few decades, especially in the areas of civil liberties and rights. Legal trends in the 1960s and 1970s tended to expand the enumerated rights of citizens in an unprecedented attempt to democratize medicine through the courts. The health rights movement—which encompassed ethnic minorities previously untreated or used as guinea pigs by hospitals, and women who advocated a return of some health care functions to midwives and other traditional caretakers—demanded an expansion of the availability of the benefits of modern medicine. Simultaneously, the individual rights of the patient in the therapeutic setting were viewed in a new way. "Patients" became "clients" with a contractual or partnership-like participation in health care decisions.[1] Greater attention to the rights of prisoners, institutionalized persons, and the unsuspecting patient in experimental situations gave rise to an increased concern about the ethics of medical research. Ironically, as more disenfranchised people sought access to the marvels of scientific medicine, the industry was unmasked as an inhuman, bureaucratic empire. The emperor had no clothes, but that did not stop the health rights movements and legal courtesans from going for every piece of flesh they could get their hands on.

Both the left and the right were out for blood, although their concerns were oddly distorted opposites. The right decried an industry too liberal to approve heroic, lifesaving efforts and baby-saving machines that looked like the worst of brave new world, while it opposed access to routine procedures like birth control, abortion, STD prevention education, even nutrition programs. Their lawyers geared up to protect the rights of the unborn and infants whose only chance was baboon heart transplants in relatively uncontrolled (by medical standards) settings, while they attacked straightforward civil measures designed to allow individuals to make simple decisions about their own bodily care.

The left, women's movement, and gay health movement, on the other hand, attacked an industry that was inaccessible to community participation and that prioritized expensive, highly technological therapies over simple, holistic measures. Their lawyers sought to reverse the prejudices against minorities that were embedded in medical terms and practices, and to legislate greater individual choice and participation.

By the 1970s, the medical industry became willy-nilly the site of struggle over political and social issues that were not always directly medical, and often couched in terms that were not overtly oppositional. Only in rare cases, such as abortion, were medical professionals required to decide where to throw their support. In most cases, the medical establishment was busy worrying about cost containment, as more people demanded services while federal and third party support drew tighter fiscal limits. The demasking of modern medicine and the embarrassing admission that fiscal managers played some of the key roles in the healing profession's choices led to what Starr calls a "therapeutic nihilism."[2] Where once medicine was given credit for advances that were more properly due to urban planning, sanitation engineering, and the educational projects of communities concerned with nutritional and public health, in the 1970s medicine got no credit, even when it was due.

The U.S. entered the era of AIDS with conflicting demands: enormous cynicism surrounded the very enterprise of medicine, costs were thought to be too high, and medicine was alternately believed to have caused oppression by inappropriately labeling people and to have helped relieve some oppression by pronouncing blacks the biological equals of whites, admitting that women's reproductive anatomy is compatible with work, and that homosexuality is a "normal" difference, not a biological defect. The arrival of AIDS provoked even more contradictory demands from both the left and the right. Rightists claimed that any money spent on AIDS was too much, that AIDS was an elective disease created by homosexuals who might just as well die off. Lesbian and gay activists demanded more responsive funding, and more concerted research, but cautioned their brothers not to get involved in the research until legal issues could be sorted out.

AIDS caused a legal crisis as well as a medical one, as patients suffered bad treatment, research subjects discovered the catch-22 in the fine print, and lesbians/gay men were subjected to renewed discrimination. The legal problems of the several at-risk communities multiply, since illegal Haitian immigrants, lesbians/gay men, and intravenous drug users are already in legal jeopardy.

## Family law meets the gay couple (and friends)

The legal issues of AIDS begin with the legally mundane but intensely personal matters of wills and power to make medical decisions for lovers. These legal issues arose first, since it was some time before the broader political dimensions of AIDS took shape. Many gay and gay-sensitive attorneys set to work designing functional wills and power of attorney or power of appointment documents which would enable lovers or close, caretaking friends of people with AIDS (PWAs) to do business for them when they were unable to go to the bank or needed assistance in making medical decisions.

Both of these areas of law had already experienced important inroads by lesbian/gay activists, but wills made in favor of lovers continue to meet challenge by biological relatives of the deceased. AIDS support workers tell horror stories of families, often long estranged, who appear on the scene during the late stages of a PWA's progress, or sometimes only after her or his death. They enter a developed network of care and support with the attitude that "Mom/Dad is here now, the rest of you can go home." Families attempt to take control over the therapeutic decision-making and management of the estate that have been handed over to lovers, friends, or designated support volunteers.

The broad social stereotype that lesbian/gay people lead shallow, lonely lives does not recognize the ways in which friendship networks, lovers, and community organizations are coping with the needs of sons, daughters, brothers, sisters, husbands, or wives with AIDS. The strong feelings of ambivalence toward the institution of the family in general and often toward particular family members make the PWA very susceptible to family demands, creating angry feelings and unclear roles in the already tense hospital setting.

Fortunately, some doctors have become sensitive to the importance for the patient of having his or her lovers, friends, and volunteer support team treated equally with the traditional family. In less progressive communities, or in cases where a gay man has been closeted, tremendous friction occurs in the decision-making process at the hospital and in the disposition of the belongings of the deceased person. Hospice workers and lovers have been accused of tricking the sick person for their own gain, and of attempting to steal the belongings of the PWA. Even the support organizations have occasionally been challenged by angry relatives when people with AIDS have made wills in favor of the non-profit entity that has supported them in their illness. Certainly, no one would even think of accusing Catholic Charities, Inc. or the Salvation Army of such crass self-interest in providing a safety net for the disenfranchised or needy, but the stereotypes of gay men and the lesbian/gay community make it easy to ignore the real commitment and love that have gone into each situation of supporting a person with AIDS. The wheels of justice are often kicked into place at the very moment when the people who have spent so much of their time with the PWA need a chance to reflect and recover, as well as some recognition of what they have experienced in the midst of a hostile or indifferent society that is nowhere prepared to cope with AIDS. Although they are seemingly simple documents, wills and powers of attorney have provided some of the nastiest legal encounters in the AIDS crisis.

## Getting a little service from the less than completely helping professions

Hot on the heels of those people who had encountered a rough trail after the hospital were the people who were trying to get in to be cared for. Once it was clear that AIDS was actually an epidemic and not just a collection of cases, emergency care personnel, dentists, hospital support services, doctors and nurses, even undertakers began refusing to get anywhere near a person with AIDS. AIDS presented an unforeseen case for medical workers who had grown up and been trained in an age that did not know the constant threat of contracting a deadly illness in their line of work. Other than occasional, isolated cases, most hospital workers only feared contracting hepatitis or tuberculosis, which might cause a short-term illness, but would rarely be fatal. AIDS created a serious crisis in medical care delivery ethics: the image of the tireless and self-sacrificing nurse, doctor, ambulance attendant, or emergency room attendant quickly gave way as workers consulted with their union representatives and refused to treat patients. Although hospitals and professional associations have developed precautions for handling AIDS cases, many workers simply do not believe the protocols are adequate. Each new medical discovery reopens the contagion question. As long as the researchers can provide data that hospital workers who follow precautions do not increase their chances of getting AIDS, the legal and ethical establishments back up the right of the patient. What happens, however, when a health care worker *does* get AIDS at the job? Which way will justice wink then?

The conservative police and prison guard unions continue to maintain that they should not be forced to work with people who might even be suspected of having ("harboring" is the term they generally use) AIDS.[3] The lack of any clear knowledge about who has or might be at risk for AIDS made it immediately evident that these elective injunctions could be construed to include anyone who even *looked* gay, Haitian, or like a prostitute or drug user. Although the medical professionals have uneasily gone back on the job, there are still occasional stories of indigent people left untreated or AIDS patients in hospitals left for several shifts lying in their full bedpans, having their food left at the door, or being shipped off to other care facilities.

A California lawyer is currently suing the city of Los Angeles because paramedics under its jurisdiction failed to touch or assist him when he suffered a heart attack. The attendants refused to treat him, incorrectly believing that he had AIDS. The suit for $1 million is now in Los Angeles County Superior Court.[4]

A man with AIDS who stood trial for a stabbing incident got a taste of "guilty until proven innocent," as prospective jurors were told that the defendant had AIDS. Although jurors were assured that they could not catch the disease by simply being in the courtroom, they were allowed to step down if they feared contracting the disease. Despite doctors' assurances, the defendant and the court marshalls wore surgical masks and gowns. Of course, AIDS was completely irrelevant to the prosecution's case. Even blind justice must have gone home weary after such an obvious, symbolic display of the defendant's "guilt" before the trial had even begun.[5]

Lesbian/gay rights advocates and lawyers set to work, often behind the scenes, to make sure that workers used the precautions dictated by their professional associations. There were two lines of attack used to insure access to services: existing civil rights statutes that included sexual preference, and existing disability laws.

New York City, which has taken a lead in AIDS-related legal and legislative measures, includes sexual orientation under its equal access clauses. The city and state human rights commissions include people with AIDS within the scope of disability and handicap provisions, and both extend disability statutes to those perceived to have a physical, mental, or medical disability. Although both avenues of equal access arguments are open, the sexual orientation segment of access to municipal hospitals does not have a clear mechanism for redress.[6]

Regulations governing hospital admissions vary, but, in general, public hospitals are required to treat patients in immediate need of services without questioning their ability to pay. However, hospitals do not necessarily have to admit everyone who walks in, and may go through a review and admission process. There are no clear-cut standards for admission, especially with a relatively new illness like AIDS where possible outcomes are not well known.

Since AIDS is so new, doctors must continually make judgment calls without solid guidelines. There are no established protocols to tell a doctor that, for example, a person experiencing a sudden worsening of PCP in the middle of the night requires admission in a high or low number of instances. Doctors must rely on their experience (which is often non-existent in the case of AIDS) and their self-education (which may be minimal). This leaves a tremendous margin of prejudice, fear, and ignorance to color an admitting physician's decisions. Although many of the major hospitals that handle a higher number of AIDS patients have instituted hospital-wide orientation programs about AIDS, the transience of interns makes it difficult to reach every employee and to pin down hospitals on their enacted policy.

The lack of care protocols, especially in emergency situations surrounding AIDS, creates a second difficulty. It may be more difficult to prove improper care unless there is absolutely clear evidence that a particular course adversely affected the patient. Doctors have traditionally been disinclined to testify against one another, and the more a case relies on gray areas of judgment, the more unwilling doctors are to comment negatively on a colleague's performance. In addition, stereotyping of gay men as hysterical may predispose those listening to their late-night complaints to view their distress as related to their sexual orientation rather than to the complex and often dramatic symptoms that signal a medical crisis in a PWA.

People with AIDS have also encountered difficulty in claiming public benefits, such as SSI and SSA, food stamps, or fuel assistance. AIDS has heavily taxed the public benefits systems in the large cities with a high incidence of the disease, but the problem extends beyond mere numbers. AIDS strikes a previously healthy and quite young population, while many of the public assistance programs are predicated on covering chronic illnesses or disabilities associated with aging. An estimated 40 to 60 percent of the people with AIDS are un- or underinsured for this type of illness and must seek public assistance to cover their medical care. This creates an additional reason to fear job loss if one's homosexuality or AIDS diagnosis becomes known: the insurance benefits extended by the employer may be the only recourse for a person with AIDS. This is particularly a problem for military personnel, who may be discharged if their homosexuality becomes known. Thus, military men who have AIDS may be extremely reluctant to admit to homosexual behavior or intravenous drug use. The recent Dronenburg case in the Washington, D.C. area provided another reason to fear expulsion from the military, since the courts (under Justice Bork, a probable Supreme Court appointee under Reagan) held that the right to privacy does not extend to homosexuals employed by the government.

Legal advocates have had to use pressure to get AIDS, and later AIDS-Related Complex (ARC), classified as a disability under SSI, SSA, and other program guidelines. These programs are complicated and difficult to apply for under ordinary circumstances, but in the case of AIDS/ARC, with their wide range of clinical manifestations and unusual age distribution, even entering the system can seem insurmountable. Often, applications are turned down and must be appealed, resulting in lost time and the need for expert assistance. AIDS organizations in the larger cities provide technical assistance by social workers experienced in maneuvering their clients through the maze of welfare programs. In addition, considerable efforts at education and negotiation go on behind the scenes to update the various programs' formulas to be responsive to changing needs.

Intravenous drug users, prostitutes, and Haitians with AIDS face additional problems in obtaining benefits since they live in legal limbo. Some of the affected Haitians are in this country illegally and fear deportation if they make any appearance in a government office. Prostitutes and IV drug users have experienced a history of harassment by these very government agencies and may fear legal reprisal or just plain indifference. Intravenous drug users who are on methadone maintenance programs may also fear jeopardizing their relationship to their clinic if their AIDS diagnosis becomes known when they apply for public assistance. Even more than gay men, at least in urban areas, the IV drug and prostitution subcultures and illegal entrants fear anything that makes them visible to government agencies.

Housing law has also come into play. People have been evicted because they were suspected of having AIDS or simply because they were gay. Very few municipalities have housing discrimination codes that cover sexual preference. Perhaps the most spectacular housing case involved the eviction of a New York City doctor whose practice included a number of people with AIDS. Although the doctor and his patients got an injunction against the tenants seeking to evict him, the tenants have appealed.[7]

## Law and justice

Law works by precedent through a hierarchy of courts whose opinions carry increasing weight. Change in the law occurs by a continual testing of the waters and tiny revisions based on previous decisions. Rarely does one case completely change the system of laws; rather, a whole set of smaller cases paves the way for a new decision. Legal philosophy does change, and lawyers with innovative ideas and judges sitting in key courts can speed up the process of change by findings that reflect new constitutional theories. Unfortunately, AIDS has arisen in a time when the novel changes are usually rightist in origin and when many of the influential courts are not inclined to extend civil rights to new groups.

The civil rights gains of the last few decades were in part due to one of the most liberal Supreme Courts in U.S. history. The lifetime tenure of these appointments means that one can expect a certain hue to persist long beyond the administration which appointed the particular judges. Progressives who came of age in the last thirty years have a certain optimism about the possibility of pursuing civil rights through the courts that may soon be a thing of the past. It is important to remember that the landmark cases—Brown vs. Board of Education, for example, or Roe vs. Wade—overturned decades or more of laws and precedents mandating separate but equal facilities for blacks (established as legal in 1896 in Plessy vs. Ferguson) and outlawing abortion. Laws denying women's right to vote took years to reverse and even then only through a constitutional amendment. The *philosophy* of equal rights for women has still not won an amendment even though there is case law and legislation that goes far toward extending rights to women.

When one considers the layers of legislation, lawsuits, and extra-legal murmurings—sometimes of a violent nature—lay folk are forced to conclude that "the law" works in capricious and mysterious ways indeed, and on a timetable entirely out of synch with their daily lives.

And yet, it is to the law that one must often look for remedy from discrimination or abuse.

## Medical ethics

The very emergence of biomedical ethics in the last thirty years is symptomatic of an important shift in social views of the scientific enterprise. Nazi experimentation on Jews, Gypsies, and others confined in concentration camps dramatized for the public the question of whether doctors and researchers really had society's and the individual's best interests in mind. For the first time in the history of scientific medicine, the issue of individual rights versus the public good was weighed in evaluating the methods of researchers. Before World War II's revelation of Nazi atrocities, the presumption had been that medical doctors were interested in saving lives and improving the quality of life. By virtue of their calling, they would promote the good of individual patients or research subjects and pursue the common good of increased understanding of sickness and health. The horror of the worthless, cruel, and forced Nazi experimentation—combined with the emergence of the nuclear bomb as a Damoclean threat—forced a traditionally optimistic and technocratic Western consciousness to question the ultimate good of science at all. The illusion of prosperity and improvement wrought by science, though employed for the benefit of select groups, had now to be weighed against the methods of science as well as the potential for applying science toward evil purposes.

The emergence of the image of the mad scientist in mass art forms, especially film, signalled a new era in society's contemplation of the possibilities of science. The mad scientist is the embodiment of science and technology in the pursuit of evil. These sinister figures were almost always men, and often spoke with German accents—and later Russian—and paradoxically hinted at Semitic origins as well. (The U.S. never quite came to grips with what had happened in Germany, nor fully understood that U.S. anti-Semitism was so entrenched that Jews themselves had to be blamed for their experience at the hands of the Nazis.) Women are rarely portrayed as mad scientists; the evil women inspire is corporeal, sexual. When women are mad scientists, they are always dark foreigners whose hyper-rationality robs them of any sexuality or positive feminine qualities.

The vast, overt, and unself-consciously racist Nazi enterprise masked the fact that very similar experiments had been and continue to be conducted in the U.S. on rural blacks, behind the closed doors of prisons, on retarded citizens, and on poor, third world clients of city teaching hospitals.[8] The code of medical ethics formulated after the Nuremburg trials, where Nazi scientists were sentenced to death by hanging, was never fully implemented in the U.S.[9] Trade secrets laws protect pharmaceutical companies from scrutiny of their research, permitting less scrupulous researchers to hide behind lawyers, as in the case of toxic shock. The World Health Organization of the United Nations has consistently criticized U.S. research policies, bluntly challenging the idea that the U.S. is the most civilized and scientifically advanced country in the world.

Attempts at regulating research, even when trade secrets and patent laws do not impede ethical conduct, are based on unrealistic ideas about the ability of minorities to participate fully as citizens under the law. Minorities—people considered not quite human by dint of some difference—are not always adequately protected under medical ethics guidelines because society does not evenly distribute rights and protections. The idea of "informed consent" rests on assumptions about who can consent, and under what circumstances, that do not take into account the subtle and obvious ways in which minority people may be forced to trade rights for protection. Virtually any medical researcher who is so inclined could claim to have obtained the informed consent— a signed contract—of a person who, because of some kind of disadvantage, might not be considered by an ethicist to have fully understood the effect of her or his consent. People may be permitted to consent who lack the knowledge, resources, or ability to act publicly in order to seek redress if their rights are violated. Prisoners, for example, do not always have a clear picture of their rights (and neither do the courts) and are particularly vulnerable to coercion in an experimental setting. Free and fully acting citizens may also have difficulty weighing choices about consent. If there are cultural differences, as in the classic travesty of the Tuskegee project, researchers may inadequately or erroneously explain what they are doing, resulting in less than informed consent and ultimately compromising the validity of the research, since participants could not reasonably have complied with protocols.[10]

Ethically, consent must be based in part on an altruistic desire to aid in scientific discovery of potential benefit to others. If incentives are used, they must not be so great as to encourage people to consent against their best interests. In addition, the possibilities of actually learning something of value in the project must be clear, or a researcher is asking a participant to make some sacrifice of time or risk some harm for no constructive end. When researchers submit proposals for consideration, the research design's ability to actually produce informative results is weighed very heavily in a decision on the project.[11]

In the case of AIDS, the very fact of experiencing a life-threatening disease with no known cause or cure tips the balance of informed consent, especially in therapeutic trials. If the alternatives are almost certain death versus possible death with experimental treatment, it is as difficult to feel wholly satisfied with consent as it would be difficult to withhold a possibly beneficial experimental drug. Certainly, cancer researchers have long faced this very problem. Sadly, the record on cancer "cures" makes one cynical about embarking on therapeutic trial studies. Therapeutic trials must insure consent, confidentiality, and follow-up if remedies, effective tests, or vaccines are found.

The new medical and old social problems raised by AIDS research—and the lesbian and gay community's ability to resist abuse— have cast the legal and ethical theorists guiding human subject research into a quandary. The problems triggered by the appearance of a deadly, apparently communicable disease closely associated with stigmatized groups, motivated the Hastings Center Institute of Society, Ethics, and the Life Sciences to undertake a clarification of guidelines specifically for research on AIDS.[12] But they too stumbled over the unique problems presented by AIDS, in the conflicting demands of research, surveillance, and the need for therapies.

Medical research and public health concerns have converged before, perhaps most notoriously in the venereal disease projects from World War I to the present. (The Tuskegee studies were exposed in the 1970s, and Alan Brandt's new book *No Magic Bullets* suggests surveillance of prostitutes should be more widely examined.)[13] The problems encountered in obtaining accurate information in VD control projects in the past compelled AIDS researchers to insure some level of confidentiality if they were to get compliance from those interviewed. The Hastings Center report notes:

> Unless they have confidence in the systems designed to protect their privacy and in the people to whom personal information is entrusted, they will face a difficult choice: either to provide inaccurate or incomplete data, thus compromising the validity of the research, or to give accurate and full data, thus placing themselves at risk.[14]

For a closeted gay man with a wife, family, or job he cannot lose, it is far easier to claim to have contracted AIDS from a prostitute than to admit to being homosexual. Not only does such a false claim create research and confidentiality problems, but it also fuels the anti-gay fires while appearing to add evidence that AIDS can and will inevitably seep out into the "general population."

The whole idea of confidence in the medical profession is particularly problematic in the political climate of the 1980s, which have seen a shift away from national concern about civil rights and toward a conservativism that trades in hatred of lesbians/gay men, prostitutes, blacks, drug users. The health radicalism of the 1960s, which had sought to extend the apparent benefits of modern medicine to the previously disenfranchised, led to a general cynicism about the efficacy of medicine: it had found no cure for cancer and the overall health of Americans had declined in spite (or, some would charge, because) of the highly touted technologies of the health care industry. The 1970s saw a further increase in suspicion and hostility toward doctors, as lawyers, ethicists, and liberal activists increasingly stepped in to protect clients from the now-defrocked medical empire. Illich and others claimed that clinical medicine actually caused more disease and death than it cured, and iatrogenic disease (illness caused by doctors) became a popular topic of journalists and health activists—especially death or further complications caused by new drugs or expensive therapies.[15]

In addition to this general erosion of confidence in the medical profession, many citizens and clinicians had serious reservations about the quality of care available in the average city hospital. Hospitals had begun to evolve into teaching institutions in the late 1800s, as the method of clinical observation shifted away from the sick individual and toward the comparison of many cases. In urban areas, the charity hospital provided a wealth of chronic disease and ill health, and patients quickly discovered that they could become guinea pigs at the hour of their greatest distress. The hospital client remains an involuntary vehicle for medical instruction, and the seeds of the idea of clinical research are planted during the young medical student's stint in the hospital as an intern observing patients. The emphasis on seeing as wide a range of pathology as possible in this learning period (rather than the earlier notion of learning as much as possible about the complexity of disease in the individual patient) begins the process of dehumanizing the client that can eventually develop into a belief that the benefits of aggregate knowledge are more important than respect (personal or legal) for the individual client. Once doctors see cases and not people, the social stereotypes they may have will make them less likely to respond to special problems faced by their clients in legal or social jeopardy.

The Hastings Center is quite right, if dissonant with the new conservatism, in seeing part of the ethical problem in AIDS as a social one: "as a society we must express our moral commitment to the principle that all persons are due a full measure of compassion and respect." Though a bit naive, they rightly see that the people at risk for AIDS will not approach the medical system or its research arms with much trust, and have a well developed interest in less than full compliance. It is not enough for doctors to express the wish to protect their clients or subjects. The doctor or researcher must be prohibited *by law* from releasing names without good reason. And those reasons must be spelled out clearly, lest a doctor balance the common good against the individual's rights without full understanding of the social, political, and legal ramifications of doing so. In addition, the researcher must have a reasonable assurance that she/he will not be subjected to government or other harassment, as from insurance companies or employers. Some suggest that medical professionals go a step further in their exhibition of "goodwill": they should publicly support policies, such as civil rights measures, that will improve their subjects' ability to pursue legal remedies and free them from social stigma. Only when lesbians/gay people, Haitians, drug users, and prostitutes no longer fear legal or social reprisal can informed consent, confidentiality, and accurate information be assured.[16]

Some people consider the fear of government subpoena of names and medical information to be sheer paranoia, but both Hastings and Lambda Legal Defense address just that possibility. There is no standard set of case law to deal with the problem of confidentiality, since public health laws are by and large left to each state to administer. But with an increasingly conservative Supreme and District Court judgeship, and the rise of rightist legal theorists who propose far more restrictive constitutional theories, it seems reasonable to imagine the worst possibilities. Hastings suggests that a clear and consistent policy of confidentiality will stand an institution in a better light in court than a less thought out rationale. But if gay researchers or institutions ultimately refuse to comply with subpoenas, this might as easily be taken as contempt. Lesbian/gay rights are not protected or widely respected enough for individual gay rights to hold up against the ominous "public good."

In addition to concerns about willful, malicious, accidental, or subpoenaed release of subject information, subjects experience heightened anxiety about entering research at all. The emotional experience of research subjects has become a special area of concern in the case of AIDS.

## Confidentiality

There is good reason for paranoia on the part of all the people who have AIDS or who belong to the groups at risk: all are to some degree in violation of law. Homosexuality is illegal in most states; many of the Haitians are illegal entrants to the U.S. and face deportation; and intravenous drug use or ownership of drug injection apparatus is generally illegal. In addition, early in the AIDS epidemic, the Centers for Disease Control several times supplied the names of people with AIDS to other agencies, once by accident.[17] It was clear by the summer of 1983 that the CDC had not taken adequate precautions to insure the confidentiality of those people under its surveillance. New York, which because of its large number of AIDS cases and existing lesbian/gay rights organizations—especially Lambda Legal Defense and the National Gay Task Force—was first in responding to the legal aspects of the AIDS crisis, immediately passed legislation designed to protect people with AIDS, and others at risk or involved in research projects, from disclosure.[18]

The failure to insure adequate confidentiality measures has many possible consequences. On the most distressing and basic human level, people who need medical treatment may be afraid of going to doctors for fear that their illegal or stigmatized status may become known. While this may vary among those in the major affected groups—gay or bisexual men in the urban gay ghettos, men who have access to gay-sensitive health care and the legal resources of the lesbian/gay community—it is certainly an important factor affecting the decision to seek health care by Haitians and IV drug users.

AIDS became a reportable disease in most states by 1983, placing doctors in jeopardy of legal restraint if they failed to report the disease, and bringing at-risk groups more solidly under the surveillance of the Public Health Service and state public health departments. Many public health officials recognized the need to protect clients' confidentiality if they were to get good compliance. They realized that an early concern over the issue of confidentiality would inspire confidence in their protocols and increase the likelihood that healthy but exposed people would voluntarily seek screening or vaccination if they become available. However, government agencies have not been cognizant of the additional concerns of people in risk groups, and have overlooked the past history of abuse of confidentiality and disregard for the special concerns these people have in seeking medical care.

With the increasing right-wing backlash accelerated by AIDS's connection with homosexuality, the penalties for risking exposure as a homosexual increase as a factor in the individual's willingness to seek appropriate medical assistance. The stereotype of gay men as irresponsible and self-destructive has also resulted in the presumption by public health officials that the lesbian/gay community will not cooperate in sex education or voluntarily stop donating blood. Although the medical establishment has in some ways learned that it must cooperate with gay organizations, the bias against considering gay men as cooperative increases in direct proportion to beliefs about their promiscuity. Like the social ideas about sexual behavior, there is a wide, if not always articulated belief, that gay men will not cooperate in attempts to alter their sexual behavior, with no understanding about how the gay male sexual community functions or what messages have been conveyed by the government in the past.

In reality, the lesbian/gay community has launched massive and sensitive educational campaigns about "safe sex," but sex education is so discouraged in this country that several states have considered them insufficient and have begun to make moves toward exercising public health prerogatives to quarantine people with AIDS or establish legal penalties against homosexual acts. California submitted its public health statutes to lawyers, and shortly after that closed all establishments in San Francisco that were believed to have sex on the premises. The bars, baths, and bookstores were allowed to reopen only if they enforced the safe sex guidelines established by a local AIDS organization. Each establishment was required to hire staff to make frequent rounds, and had to insure that a ratio of surveillance staff to clients was maintained.

When faced with the choice of improbable but possible exposure to AIDS versus an almost certain harm resulting from admitting to being gay, it is not surprising that a healthy gay man might reasonably decide not to go to the doctor for screening. For bisexual men whose homosexual activity is hidden, or for gay men who live in smaller towns or regions where homosexuality is highly stigmatized or illegal, the equation tips even further against going to a doctor. A paradoxical corollary applies to this concern about the relative harm of coming out versus finding out about AIDS: with the equivocal HTLV-III blood test, openly gay men, who are unaware of the legal or insurance problems a positive test might cause, may rush out to get tested as soon as the test becomes widely available. The lesbian/gay community will experience a widespread and uncontrollable reaction to test results in individuals, as well as possible inter-community tensions which federal agencies may be able to manipulate to their advantage. As AIDS becomes more prevalent outside the urban gay male community, the many different needs of gay men in other living situations may create conditions where legal strategies are undermined by lack of cooperation of gay men who do not understand or are not aware of their civil rights. The great number of false positives from widespread HTLV-III antibody testing may also create a large pool of "straight," low risk people with even more contradictory concerns.

Privacy and civil rights law has tended, under the influence of the new left, feminist, and lesbian/gay movements, to become more inclusive, to extend to categories of people or activities that were not necessarily originally enumerated. As the political climate shifts, however, and the composition of the Supreme Court changes, there is even greater reason to fear that lists originally procured and protected with the best of intentions may later become weapons against disenfranchised groups. The general social concern expressed about AIDS outside the affected groups is not motivated by a desire to help the homosexual, Haitian, IV drug user, or prostitute—as might have been argued in more liberal times, in spite of a tacit moral sentiment against these people—but to protect the "innocent" victims, allegedly including straight men with no risk other than going to prostitutes, from the social deviants who middle Americans believe "produced" AIDS.

No one in U.S. society has ever been fully equal under the law, fully innocent until proven guilty, especially when public health is balanced against individual liberties. In the current political climate, where abortion rights, First Amendment rights, and the whole notion of a right to privacy (who needs to be private unless they are doing something bad?) are under attack, there is no pretense that anyone other than traditional, god-fearing, Christian family members deserves equal treatment under the law. The equation promoting the common good is weighted unapologetically against lesbians/gay men, liberated women, third world people, and anything liberal. In a system that says gay men should sacrifice a little freedom to the Public Health Service to produce a greater social good, the lives saved through faithful and well-intentioned cooperation with AIDS surveillance and research will not and may not be intended to be those whose lives are at risk.

# 7.

# The New Right

At the beginning of its emergence in the 1970s, the new right's social program seemed sadly out of step with the times. Although their economic agenda has received extensive analysis and strategic attention, many progressives view the new right's regressive social agenda as a smoke screen to be taken seriously only as a *bas relief* of the reactionary spirit hidden among more sophisticated conservatives. But to dismiss the absurdity of new right rhetoric misses the real power that their visceral authoritarianism holds on a profoundly Calvinist nation.

The new right's response to AIDS displays in blatant, ghastly terms what is latent in even the most sophisticated liberals. Old notions of sin, sickness, and criminality emerge in a full program aimed at suppressing difference. Skeptical that scientific "facts" are part of a liberal conspiracy, radical rightists look for physical signs that distinguish the sinful from the pure. One of the remarkable features of fundamentalist Christian and neo-populist right-wing ideologues is their obsession with matters corporeal. In ironic contrast, the U.S. left has in recent years been more fascinated by intellectual and historical processes. This political mind/body split creates an almost unbridgeable conceptual gulf laying each open to humorous and vicious caricature in the literature of the other.

Physical control and restraint are ideologically, strategically, and symbolically significant to the new right. Eras of rightist ascendancy are marked by legislative shifts toward more stringent physical controls—law and order, capital punishment, punishment of sexuality, more stringent pedagogical styles. Rightist ascendancy is accompanied by renewed interest in participation in organized religion, with its individual daily rituals of discipline, and its weekly collective worship.[1]

A symbolism of physical restraint and bodily invasion translates the abstract Calvinist concepts of the right-wing ideology into a vivid and visceral reality, deeply felt by adherents and opponents alike. Using lurid descriptions and hateful edicts, propagandists ask their constituencies whether they want to expose their children to the sin and sickness of homosexuals, blacks, Jews, even "idol worshiping" Catholics. Implicit in their rhetoric, and explicit in their policies, is a notion of racial purity and absolute community consensus that decries pluralism and abhors "mixing."

### See no evil

A political ideology that taps deep, inchoate feelings about pain and pleasure, freedom and restraint has particular potency. Profoundly morbid, yet sincerely apocalyptic, the right-wing populism terrifies individuals with stories of plots barely held in check by rituals of cleansing and constant vigilance to avert one's eyes lest one inadvertently stare pure evil in the face. Although they have gained political prominence with rhetoric about the return to traditional norms, the new right is a profoundly counter-cultural movement: like the apocalyptic left movement of the 1960s, their goal is to supplant the existing culture.

Calvinism's bizarre mix of predestination with scrutiny of acts as signs of election loses little of its paranoid force and zealotry through secularization and technocratization. Indeed, these trends reignite the Calvinist search for proof of God's supremacy over "man."[2] New right Calvinism accedes to a program of "Christ against culture" by allowing leaders to prove their election in symbolic or real battle with the evil forces of homosexuality, abortion, miscegenation, etc.[3]

Their crude mix of crusading authoritarianism and religious populism allows new right leaders to go out and do battle with the forces of perversion, sparing the innocent citizen the danger of confronting the foe him/herself. Computer-engineered direct mail and TV evangelism are the miracle of technology in the service of Calvinism. By paying money to the various groups, the vigilant moralist can stay locked safely at home, out of danger of pollution by contact with the diseased sinners.

Yet, there is a lot of peeping between the fingers. New right leaders prove their cause (and garner ever more funds) with tantalizing glimpses of the grotesque evils they are combating. But the propagandists and direct-mail letter writers must continually up the ante: each new cause must seem more lurid, more dangerous, more immediate than the last if they expect letters to get more support. It is less the particular information conveyed than the process of breaking taboos that repulses and tantalizes readers and contributors. The tactic turns product advertising on its head: instead of selling items which the consumer can't do without, the radical right markets shocking and threatening images which readers can't afford to live with.[4] A classic direct-mail fundraising letter from the American Family Association encourages its readers with a come-on to close down homosexual establishments by signing their petition:

> Dear Family Member,
> Since AIDS is transmitted primarily by perverse homosexuals, your name on my national petition to quarantine all homosexual establishments is crucial to your family's health and security...These disease carrying deviants wander the street unconcerned, possibly making *you* their next victim. What else can you expect from sex-crazed degenerates but selfishness?

Finally, after impressing the reader with the immediacy and magnitude of this threat, it is clear that only money will do the trick:

> Our effort to WIPE OUT AIDS will cost thousands of dollars. I have established a budget of $28,570.00 for the next 15 days' expenses. We must fight this crucial battle through the newspapers, television media and even door to door! But all this costs money...I urge you to return your signed petition and generous gift to me today.
> P.S. Only your contribution can help us protect Americans from the "Gay Plague" and its perverted carriers. Please send your generous contribution and signed petition to me today.[5]

Signing a petition (although they do make their way to governors and federal officials like Surgeon General Koop) is a variation on reader participation schemes: "put the enclosed token in the slot and sent $25 for your subscription to—."

Christian Family Renewal circulated a similar "petition" as a fundraiser:

> You may soon fall victim to an irreversible, fatal disease! And it won't be your fault!

> But, you'll have to pay the terrible price anyway because of
> the promiscuous homosexuals, whose lustful life-styles have
> created this uncontrollable incurable plague.

They cleverly play on the euphemism of "life-style" to equate gay
rights with destruction.

> And now, they've acquired their own distinct death-style, the
> AIDS plague, and like all their other rights, the homosexuals
> are forcing this painful, deadly disease on the rest of society.
> ...Send the largest gift you can as if your life—and it very well
> may—depended on it.
> AIDS MUST BE STOPPED NOW! I'm trusting you realize
> the drastic and emergency steps we're about to take together is
> the only way to stop this dreaded disease.[6]

Enclosed with this letter is a yellow petition and donation card that
is bordered with the purple imprint of, presumably, healthy cells.

The right's systematic misinformation and mind-boggling distor-
tion of medical reports blurs the distinction between transmission of an
etiological agent during sexual activity and the sexual acts themselves:
homosexual acts become the *prima facie* cause of AIDS. Once the
notion of a virus is dropped from the equation, the disease becomes
proof of the commission of an immoral act. Death is not too great a
penalty for violation of moral law. Conversely, for a "normal" or
"innocent" person to die as the result of this disease is a horrible
travesty, worse than the disease itself.

The ultimate corporeal threat of death or proof of election through
death is important ammunition in the arsenal of radical right hate
ideology. To die for a just cause (like war) ennobles life. To desecrate
life (by being a homosexual or having an abortion) merits death. In
Calvinist ideology, life itself is not symbolically valued except as an
opportunity to demonstrate election. Death is far more valuable as a
principle for organizing morality. Predestination means that no good
works can produce salvation, but to doubt one's election and live as if
one were destined for hell is the worst of sins. Risking death provides an
opportunity to prove election by dramatically demonstrating faith. To
rightists, some death is very cheap indeed, but life is even cheaper. The
rightists are firmly and self-consciously apocalyptic and can strategize
final solutions.

AIDS is a particularly potent symbol for the hard-line radical right
because it is evidence of sin, God's disfavor, and an ultimate solution: it
is both a sign and a punishment embodied in one of the groups targeted

for political decimation long before AIDS. Even rightist doctors, whom one supposes might separate their science and bigotry, have fused them into pseudoscientific logic:

> If we act as empirical scientists, can we not see the implications of the data before us? If homosexuality, or even just male homosexuality, is "OK," then why the high prevalence of associated complications both in general and especially with respect to AIDS? Might not these "complications" be "consequences"? Might it be that our society's approval of homosexuality is an error and that the unsubtle words of wisdom of the Bible are frightfully correct?
>
> Indeed, from an empirical medical perspective alone, current scientific observation seems to require the conclusion that homosexuality is a pathologic condition.[7]

## Speak no evil

Until very recently, those who had to make authoritative pronouncements on homosexuality used euphemisms that made it clear that "it" was not a fit topic of conversation. Numerous historians have catalogued the "namelessness" of this "crime" that sheds light on evolving social views of homosexuality. An Illinois judge was forced to comment on the subject in 1897, and said that the crime against nature was "not fit to be named among Christians."[8] D'Emilio notes that "commentators composed their remarks according to a formula that discouraged further amplification."

Through the 1950s and 1960s, although lesbian/gay activists saw some increased coverage of their issues and events, homosexuality was a topic that many wanted neither to see nor hear about. An October 7, 1959, San Francisco *Progress* headline read, "Sex Deviates Make San Francisco Headquarters." The story read, "homosexualism has been allowed to flourish to a shocking extent, and under shocking circumstances."[9] Lest the poor innocent who has never even heard of homosexualism be misled, he or she is repeatedly told that sex deviates are on the rise, and it is "shocking" but the story offers no concrete information on who these sex deviates are or what it is they do. This incipient form of social terrorism lets people know that something is happening that they are better off not knowing about. The fascist mentality that unearthed and described "spy rings" under the dubious machinations of national security invented a plot of homosexuals who were alleged to be weakening the moral fiber of U.S. citizens. Even today some rightist groups claim that homosexuality and even AIDS is a communist plot, despite the fact that communist countries and parties have generally been hostile toward homosexuality.[10] With the homosexual plot, the government and media asked citizens to trust that there was nothing of merit to know about homosexuality except that it was being vigilantly rooted out: the less said about perversion, the better.

Even after sex became accepted as a subject of scientific study with Kinsey, Masters and Johnson, Hite, Rubin, and other less popularized reports, medical doctors, religious leaders, and media still confused scientific terms and their symbolic uses. The same San Francisco *Progress* story claimed that "this unsavory wicked situation is allowed to fester and spread like a cancerous growth on the body of San Francisco." Dr. Charles Socarides, at the June 1968 AMA convention, said homosexuality was a "dread dysfunction, malignant in character, which has risen to epidemic proportions."[11]

Right-wing solipsists have used medical and military imagery interchangeably: reds and queers were alternately diseases and invasions. The military/disease imagery was honed in the 1950s during the extensively covered House Un-American Activities Committee (HUAC) trials. Although homosexuality was less overtly discussed (though much alluded to), communism and faggotry were well established as threats to U.S. security. Both were assaults from within U.S. culture— infiltration—by people who didn't look different to the untrained eye. The HUAC trials heightened the paranoid search for the telltale limp wrist or a certain turn of nose—signs of perversion or foreignness that became markers of guilt that needed no court.

Despite recent losses, the lesbian/gay community made a crucial, if little observed gain, which cannot be repealed along with civil rights statutes. Through increasing coverage of lesbian/gay issues in news and features, as well as the proliferation of lesbian/gay book titles and an aboveground press, homosexuality has acquired not only "a name," but a sophisticated vocabulary of distinctions. Language about homosexuality has evolved from vague, embarrassed references through the euphemistic "lifestyle" until today even very conservative politicians refer to the "lesbian and gay community" as they rail against homosexuality. "Lifestyle" has become appropriated from "me generation" jargon to indicate a consumerist neo-pluralism. While serving as editor of Boston's *Gay Community News*, I received a call asking for the "Lifestyle" editor. I was tempted to reply in my best high camp, "But darling, we *are* a lifestyle."

Media coverage surrounding lesbian/gay victories and losses accepts the existence of a lesbian/gay political force: a vote to be courted by liberals, a conspiracy to be unmasked by rightists. Mainstream media accounts of lesbian/gay political activity rubber stamped the consolidation of a lesbian/gay identity that has at least some political interests in common by admitting the existence of a constituency capable of collective action. In the new right literature, lesbians and gay men graduated from a covert conspiracy to an audacious and open lobby.

This more open discourse on homosexuality made possible a kind of coverage of AIDS that would have been unfathomable fifteen years ago. Not only do lesbians and gay men exist, but, at least in the AIDS coverage, they are undoubtedly sexual beings. And in a second interesting shift, the actuality of gay male sex acts has reached some level of public articulation, even if more colloquial terms like "cock sucking" or "fucking" are replaced by "oral" and "anal" intercourse. Under the guise of scientific reporting, direct references to gay male sex acts moved from crime stories buried in the Help Wanted section, to the front page of the news and "living" sections. Implicitly, the idea that scientists were examining these taboo areas of the "love that dare not speak its name" both legitimized and demythologized gay male (but not lesbian) sexual practice for at least some media consumers.

A more explicit discussion of gay male sex is necessary in the new right literature, too, if they are to capitalize on this opportunity to prove their point. Discussion of AIDS in scientific terms by right-wing doctors and lay people serves to legitimize misinformation by appearing objective and scientific while making their political agenda clear with prefaces to the "facts" that are apologies for having to tell innocent people these disgusting things. In order to cash in on the political power of science, new right propagandists must scientologize their anti-sex tracts and add the litany of gay male sex acts to counter claims that homosexuality is just another kind of sex: recitation provides a vivid expose of the "excesses" of homosexuality. It is no longer enough to allude to vague acts that "can't be named by Christians."

The laundry list of perverse acts elicits great interest among new rightists, and a constantly increasing diet seems to be necessary to feed this horror of unleashed sexuality and sex germs. The scientific discussion of heterosexual sex that has given baby boom adults a blase attitude toward imagery that shocked their parents has merely been extended to gay male sex (no one yet knows what lesbians do!). The list isn't nearly as frightening as the speak-no-evil rightists feared, even if the inflated numbers of "average" sexual partners is mind-boggling (it's just new math). The new right's own revelation of perverse sexual practices has undermined its ability to shock.

## Rightist neo-populism

The new right did not spring into existence full-blown merely to combat the evils of homosexuality and abortion, although U.S. activism is so often fragmented and ahistorical that it must seem that way to those activists who cut their teeth in the last two decades. Nor is the new right a coherent monolith.

The new right welds together bits of fundamentalist Christianity, fear of anything different, genuine frustration with leaders who don't seem to represent anyone, and a political primitivism reminiscent of the Know-Nothing Party, a similar U.S. grassroots reactionism that gained prominence in the mid-nineteenth century.

At their height, the Know-Nothings elected seventy-five congressional representatives but they never passed any significant legislation. Their appeal lay in their finger-pointing: "aliens" (European immigrants, not space invaders) were the root of all social ills. They offered no concrete solution, and supported no coherent program. Like the new right today, they became entrenched in a mentality of zealous separatism predicated on opposition to an inchoate and contradictory "other" composed of a plurality of immigrants and urbanites in the burgeoning industrialized East. The Know-Nothings are distinguished by their isolationism, populism, negativism, and attitude that the West represented the "real America." Nostalgic and anti-progressive, the Know-Nothings split over the issue of slavery, and by 1895 they had no significant federal representation and were reduced to an out-of-touch, infighting group of political incompetents.[12]

The rift between the East and the West/South bloc of "pioneers" that spawned the Know-Nothings extends for over one hundred years of U.S. political history, and lays some of the foundation for the new right today. The new Old West cowboy mentality of Reaganism provides a convenient symbol for the new right's ascendancy in the 1980s, even if Reagan did not live up to the new right's expectations in his first term by being too corporatist and centralist. Through his rhetoric of traditionalism and the sheer idiocy of his public blunders, Reagan thrives in his second term because of the zealous personality cult surrounding him. If Reagan says everyone is better off, many people are convinced, in spite of real decreases in spending power as measured by common indexes. Liberals and leftists who fail to see the power of the Calvinist undercurrent tapped by Reaganism cannot understand why economic oppression seems like moral liberation. Material conditions no longer matter to the Protestant middle and lower classes if cessation of doubt rather than worldly wealth becomes the measure of Christian election.

> It is the rich who by risking their wealth ultimately lose it, and save the economy... That is the function of the rich: fostering opportunities for the classes below them in the continuing drama of creation of wealth and progress.
> This drama is most essentially not of measurable money and machines, aggregations and distributions, but of mind and morale. [13]

With a brash wave of his wand, George Gilder, architect of Reagan's supply-side ethics, dismisses all materialist analysis and class antagonisms. The wealthy who engage in capitalism (not charity) are altruistic because they engender opportunities for the whole economy. The new southern and western rich, whose vast wealth is amassed from venture capitalist endeavors (not inheritance or trusts, like the eastern establishment wealthy) are the elect, not because to be rich is to be saved, but rather because they command and deploy the resources which, when "lost," save the whole economy. The rugged *individual* capitalist may lose his shirt by financing the wrong business, but even this proves his election: doubting capital, and not risking it, is a grave offense and these wealthy will not enter the gates of heaven. This parable of wealth and poverty, faith and doubt gives hope to the lower classes in the most crass Horatio Algeresque sense, and tricks them into believing that their natural antagonists—the financially active rich— are really trying to help them.

## The cultural battlelines

The 1970s were marked by a struggle between the new right and two new political forces: the women's liberation and lesbian/gay liberation movements. Anti-Vietnam war forces had won the letter of their battle, though not the spirit, and the "ecology" movement seemed to be the trend, even if things were not progressing very rapidly. The prevailing mainstream mentality was labeled the "me generation," which, deserved or not, became a self-fulfilling media prophecy. Traditional notions of conservative versus liberal broke down: the 1970s mainstream was held together by shared economic and personal values, not by a coherent political spirit.

The idea of the "me generation" became an effective if subtle method for diverting the struggle for civil rights and cultural autonomy that marked lesbian/gay, women's, and ethnic groups' liberation struggles. As if to prove that the U.S. had won on the domestic front, even if it had lost abroad, the "me generation" ideology pretended to have overcome the color bar by including faces of color on ads for consumer products. A propaganda of introspection could ignore surface color and class differences as long as there was a Cuisinart in the kitchen and Le Car in the garage.

"Telling it like it is" gave way to "I am what I am." Liberal born-again moderationism sought to wash away the bad taste of both the conservative conspiracy of Watergate and the radical student and black riots. The "me generation" ideology neatly embraced an offended middle class of all colors, the unregulated rich, and to some extent the urban low-income people who had moved just above poverty with social service programs that had not yet been dismantled. There was still a Great Society ethos, although the political ideology of fairness at home and peace abroad was quietly being slipped out of the practicality back door. Optimistic liberals believed that progressive changes would remain intact, that the chaos was merely a settling-in period. The right was drawing different conclusions: chaos was the problem, and progressive changes were the impediment to a strong U.S. In the 1984 national election, liberal fairness gave way to a concept of justice that told the traditionally disadvantaged to pull up their own bootstraps. Threat of war was only the most blatant form of terrorism, as random, state-supported violence reached paramilitary proportions.

Feminist and lesbian/gay activists were able to mobilize in the environment of the "me generation" ethos in part because sexism and homophobia made their self-consciousness seem like introspection, "getting in touch with feelings," self-expression or acting out—1960s counter-cultural values that were twisted and marketed in the 1970s to promote consumerism over activism. The radical right could ascend in this very same environment because their rhetoric alone translated the social upheaval of the 1960s and 1970s to bewildered, conservative, non-activist citizens.

Primarily cultural critiques, all three rejected attempts to buy off a nation struggling to place in perspective a meaningless and lost war, and a sinister and lying president. Fundamentalist Christians and populist rightists were not tantalized by decadent toys and a media that increasingly promoted a sexualized consumer aesthetic. Feminists and lesbian/gay activists were not lulled by these salves to a badly bruised U.S. Women couldn't afford the toys, and at any rate, were part of the consumer package. The lesbian/gay culture, where it existed, was circumscribed from open consumption by fear of harassment or discovery. The emerging right and the feminist and lesbian/gay movements, at least on the surface, all criticized the structure of the same institutions—family, church, sexual relations.

The battlelines were drawn dramatically between the new right and the women's and lesbian/gay liberation movements, and between blacks and radical rightists. The various movements who stood in oppositions to the radical right would eventually meander toward the "rainbow coalition," a strategically and ideologically significant realignment of the last remnants of the New Deal coalition. Moderates stood by alternately amused by the incomprehensible demands of gays and women, and repulsed by the insanity of new right disinformation. Moderates did not initially take either of the groups seriously and hedged their political bets by accommodating to both.

Jimmy Carter's election most aptly captures the spirit of the moderates in the 1970s. The Carter years were distinguished by "trying to answer the spiritual needs of a frightened Calvinist mainstream while courting the very people scaring them most."[14] Carter pacified the broad mainstream with his rhetoric of moral restoration, while failing to put the lid on Pandora's box of new cultural values. The radical right and the cultural progressives both bid for structural power in the years between Watergate/Vietnam and the first Reagan election. Liberals and moderates, perplexed by non-economistic social programs, ceded the most important turf to the new right—control over the body.

Reaganism has ripped off the language of grassroots activism from the left/feminist/gay movements and dismantled the federal support for community-based programs of the 1960s and 1970s. The right-wing majoritarianism threatens to replace liberal pluralism. Despite the experience of progressives in the last two decades, whose history created a belief that grass-roots organizing is necessarily progressive, if the roots are planted in traditional soil the movement spawned will exhibit a rightward tropism. The similarity in progressive and right-wing rhetoric stems in part from a battle to control grassroots-style organizing.

The decentralist neo-populism of the new right is different from leftists' socialist populism in strategy and theory. However, the right-wing populism, and some new versions of "left" populism, bear an important feature in common. Both move toward analyzing racism and sexism in economistic terms, even though Gilder is anti-marxian and the progressives are marxian. New rightists blame liberal economic policies for supposedly making blacks and women dependent on the welfare state, which then multiplies the oppression of women by causing the breakdown of the family. If women can strike less of a bargain in the sexual arena, they must depend on the state rather than punish errant males by coercing them into economic support through marriage.

Neo-progressive economic reductionists insist that continued attention to race *per se* only incites racial tension. They believe that great strides have been made to remove individual prejudice and citizens must move on to address structural economic barriers which prohibit blacks from gaining equal economic clout. Both neo-populisms reject the cultural pluralist values embodied in the "rainbow coalition" by asserting that given equal access to material, everyone will "be the same."[15]

## Hate rhetoric

A critical point of dissonance among rightists concerns the reformability of homosexuals. Some groups have bid for greater credibility (as more "conservative" homosexuals have "come out") by tempering their rhetoric. Christian groups have countered the criticisms of their hate-mongering by professing to love the homosexual, but hate homosexuality." This logic conveniently allows that some children might grow up to be homosexuals for reasons beyond their control—hormones, bad family experiences, lack of protection from queers—and shifts the moral burden toward "making good choices," or doing what is right in the face of a bad deal. They see two categories of homosexuals: those who try not to act on their perverse urges and those who flagrantly commit homosexual acts. These groups of new rightists seek to convert homosexuals and AIDS provides particularly fertile ground. Their logic claims that anti-gay campaigns are not bigoted but compassionate programs to help the homosexuals stop killing themselves.

> This pamphlet has been written for the benefit of heterosexuals and homosexuals alike. We believe that homosexual sex practices seriously threaten the well-being of the individual homosexual along with the well-being of our nation. Our goal is to diminish that danger for both.[16]

Like Gilder's attack on liberal society this, and other groups blame AIDS and the "spread" of homosexuality on the permissive society that allowed the lesbian/gay liberation movement to even speak its name.

> Over the last two decades, Americans have become increasingly tolerant of homosexuals and "homosexual practices." What

consenting adults did in private was of no real concern at all to many of the last several generations.

Now it turns out that homosexuals and their practices can threaten our lives, our families, our children, can influence whether or not we have elective surgery, eat in certain restaurants, visit a given city or take up a certain profession or career—all because a tiny minority flaunts its lifestyle and demands that an entire nation tolerate its diseases and grant it status as a privileged minority.[17]

The new rightists differ in their position on whether the homosexual with AIDS can relinquish "his" dangerous state of homosexuality. One group claims to be more compassionate than its farther right brethren, and purports to being committed to saving AIDS "victims" through prayer.

> I had made a silent agreement with the Lord not to wear the assigned robe, plastic gloves or any other garment required in visiting an AIDS patient....I leaned closer to him and spoke very carefully, so that he would understand my words, "Charles, this is not a judgment from God but a consequence of our past lifestyles. Different people live different lifestyles. When these are out of order with God's best for us, consequences come. All of us in this room have suffered consequences and are unworthy of God's grace...."
>
> I asked Charles if he would like us to pray with him for his healing. His answer was affirmative. I explained that there are two healings for which to pray. The first and most important was his spiritual healing.
>
> We prayed also for his physical restoration. The next day, we returned to take him the New Testament on tape to feed him spiritually. We were astounded at his physical progress in 24 hours time. His fever was down....We believe with Charles that God is in the business of restoring and making WHOLE ALL THOSE WHO ARE STRUGGLING SPIRITUALLY OR PHYSICALLY WITH SATAN'S LIES.[18]

It is unclear whether they think they have cured AIDS or homosexuality. This conflation of the "gay disease" with the gay person is persistent throughout the right's AIDS literature (and everywhere else in AIDS imagery). But this lack of clarity passes unnoticed by the right-wing audience, since their real agenda is to get rid of all homosexuals one way or another.

AIDS rhetoric merely becomes a more sophisticated anti-gay campaign that pretends to be more enlightened. The patronizing tone of the literature varies from "we told you so" to "we tried to be nice to homosexuals, but this time they've gone too far." Anti-gay AIDS literature arises from the political stalemate between far right initiatives to void progressive lesbian/gay rights ordinances and the increased numbers of lesbian/gay or supportive politicians in elective and appointive offices. The right wing views AIDS as proof that even if their rhetoric and strategy was inarticulate and not wholly effective, their logic was correct: gays are a scourge to society and to themselves.

> Prayer Focus: AIDS—That God would prevent the spread of this dreaded disease to the general public, use it to expose the depravity of homosexuality and cause those who are practicing homosexuals to repent and totally reject their detestable life style. May He have mercy and bring healing to those AIDS victims who repent and turn to Him.[19]

The Tearcatchers provide a pamphlet on counseling the gay person, maintaining that the rabid right-wing Christians have given the rest of the evangelicals a bad name.[20] By the end of the several page, well-produced pamphlet containing accurate information and good resources, however, the message is much the same: convert homosexuals from their sexual practice. This view that homosexual identity can't change but individuals can stop practicing gay sex has been maintained by a range of religious institutions, including the Catholic Church and the relatively liberal Methodists. They concede that some homosexuals can't change (then they don't have to admit defeat when the lesbian/gay person keeps having lesbian/gay sexual desire) but they can be "ministered to" by helping them live happily with celibacy. This idea embraces the homosexual individual within the church but says, kindly leave your dirty sexual habits at the door, thank you. With the advent of AIDS, even the liberal Christian has stopped to wonder: if gays themselves are advocating safe sex (which, given the level of knowledge of most middle Americans about gay sexual practice, probably sounds like celibacy or at any rate marriage) then perhaps they were right to discourage gay sex all along. AIDS, like VD historically, is viewed as willfully contracted. One rightist medical doctor said: "...a logical conclusion is that AIDS is a self-inflicted disorder for the majority of those who suffer from it."[21]

The Moral Majority began lobbying against federal AIDS funding in 1982.

> If the medical community thinks that a new drug is what is needed to combat these diseases, it is deluding itself. There is a price to pay for immorality and immoral behavior.[22]

A little more than a year later:

> Why should the taxpayers have to spend money to cure diseases
> that don't have to start in the first place? Let's help the drug
> users who want to be helped and the Haitian people. But let's let
> the homosexual community do its own research. Why should
> the American taxpayer have to bail out these perverted people?[23]

Tearcatchers disapproves of this compassionless approach. Not
only will the Moral Majority's attitude endanger the public health by
not deploying all possible resources to stop the disease, but it does not
address the "real" cause of AIDS, which they claim is promiscuity.
They still oppose homosexuality, not because it is in itself immoral,
but because it is a symptom of the crisis of masculinity wrought by the
women's movement. Shunning the homosexual in the age of AIDS is
missing out on a brilliant opportunity for evangelism to people confused by progressive political movements, a sentiment echoed in the *Be
Whole* letter cited above.

But the sex problem goes deeper, U.S. Protestantism is the heir of
the Puritan notion that there is good sex and bad sex, good violence and
bad violence. Good sex takes place in the confines of marriage and
serves to weld together the family unit through procreation, or in the
more liberal home, through the healthy display of intimacy within the
married couple. Good violence is that exercised by the state through the
military or police. The new right advocates penalizing non-marital,
non-procreative sex with just violence—capital punishment, quarantine, or simply letting unrepentant homosexuals kill themselves off
with AIDS. Right-wing populism justifies its generally pro-legitimate
violence, anti-sex stand as a secular version of religious redemption.
Gilder makes particularly insidious connections between the economy
of sex and the ideology of violence:

> The key to lower-class life in contemporary America is that unre-
> lated individuals, as the census calls them, are so numerous and
> conspicuous that they set the tone for the entire community...
> ...The lives of the poor, all too often, are governed by the
> rhythms of tension and release that characterize the sexual expe-
> rience of young single men. Because female sexuality, as it
> evolved over the millennia, is psychologically rooted in the
> bearing and nurturing of children, women have long horizons
> within their very bodies, glimpses of eternity within their
> wombs. Civilized society is dependent upon the submission of
> the short-term sexuality of young men to the extended maternal
> horizons of women. This is what happens in monogamous

marriage; the man disciplines his sexuality and extends it into the future through the womb of a woman.[24]

## New right and family ideology

The new right appeals across class lines by creating a symbol of unity that makes no overt class reference. "The family" is the galvanizing symbol of the new right, and engenders programs that aim to reverse the trends that are perceived to have attacked the nuclear family. The family so ardently defended is in reality a recent and predominantly white, middle class, Anglo-American invention, and not even the dominant pattern in the U.S. As a symbol enmeshed in a politics of paranoia, the "family" neatly defines categories of people who fall outside it as intruders, anti-American. This pro-family rhetoric allows the right to see as coherent the left, feminist, and lesbian/gay liberation movements, even though these progressive movements do not agree on a common agenda. This is the same "up-against-ness" that fueled the Know-Nothings and other anti-progressive backlashes: it is easier to define a reaction against progressive changes than to develop a coherent rightist program. Only now that the right has achieved some structural power has it been necessary to create an umbrella of theory, but this theory only rationalizes disparate reactionisms rather than building a systematic plan from a clearly articulated critique. The new left experienced similar cohesion problems in the seventies, with the positive result of the emerging "rainbow coalition" but the negative trend toward a pro-family left faction and economistic neo-progressives who ignore cultural and sexual oppression.

Family rhetoric is potent and sensational, like pictures of children and puppies, and it is difficult to argue against the paranoid clutching for something that is more myth than reality. Major rightist efforts have attempted to legislate a pro-family agenda. The Family Protection Act, now being re-submitted to congress in pieces, as well as the outrageous Model Sexuality Bill (which appears in piecemeal form as an exclusion of other fair practice bills) reverse legislation which enabled greater access to social services and civil rights remedies for a wide range of people.[25] These bills recreate the pre-civil rights structural impediments, only this time through a conscious effort.

## Women and the right

The new right updates the script of traditional gender-based social disparity. Men are still out riding the political range, risking contact with the pagan perverts while fighting for gun ownership, national defense, law and order. New right women protect the hearth and home through domestic politics—issues involving family, children, school, and the church. There is no contradiction between their belief that "a woman's place is in the home," and their brand of activism—women engage in public politics only on issues that are an extension of the domestic arena. The division of political labor by sex doubles the available "manpower" without creating internal splits like those experienced on the left: for example, progressive feminists organized autonomously from men after their experiences with the male dominated left.

Phyllis Schlafly, whose pamphlet "AIDS-ERA" epitomizes the new right tendency toward disinformation, claims to be a single issue leader. By subsuming abortion, lesbianism, the draft, and now AIDS under the banner of anti-ERA organizing, she claims interest in a "single issue," not a broader political (i.e. male) agenda which might, incidentally, make Schlafly's bid for power contradict her position on the ERA. Many members of her Eagle Forum disagree on the issues related to ERA but the fervor of Schlafly's rhetoric and tidy conflation prevents issue differences from emerging vocally enough to cause a split on the symbolic main issue of the ERA.[26]

The new right obscures the political agenda of the principal leaders by maintaining this illusion of grass-roots, single issue organizing. One of the major factors that has permitted the far right to maintain this position is a small core of power-brokers and several computers. Where the left has traditionally instilled a sense of political participation through direct action, the far right creates a sense of belonging and action through letter writing, petition, and financial contribution—methods that create a sense of unity and mass without gathering people together in face to face discussion. The core new right activists amass great financial resources and provoke very little opposition or call for accountability. The newsletters depend on a personal anti-intellectual style that claims its authenticity by fueling the paranoia that no one else will tell the reader the truth.[27] This intimate experience of receiving the privileged truth at home creates a zeal which requires very little commitment of time and energy, and doesn't require the new right masses to be politically active in a world full of dangerous people. This separatist ethos heightens individual paranoia and makes new right followers increasingly dependent on their leaders.

The new right has been successful in building a base of power outside big business and the two parties, traditional sources of conservative power. From their extra-party base, they have taken over the ultra-conservative wings of both parties. They promote a politics of revenge, often attacking candidates they don't like rather than offering of their own. This negative strategy allows them to rally voters against candidates who favor specific issues without having to form a coalition that can agree on enough issues to elect an alternative candidate. Issues are highlighted in a domino theory format: rightists often support candidates who have the correct view on a few key issues (especially abortion, busing, and homosexuality) but have a totally different philosophy. The new right leaders that emerge maintain an air of reluctance, and claim to be "out front followers."[28]

The differences in the various new right group's positions on AIDS create little conflict: the real goal is to manipulate AIDS to gain popular support. In decentralist rhetoric of community control or community standards, the community defined by the right excludes the people to be controlled by the standards. Thus, U.S. Department of Health and Human Services secretary, Margaret Heckler, can have it both ways when she claims that AIDS is her department's number one priority. Uncritical progressives may applaud the apparent deployment of federal resources (however scant), but the right knows that the money is going to develop blood tests and vaccines to protect "the innocent," and not primarily toward curing the sick.

# SECTION THREE
# Eros Lost and Eros Regained

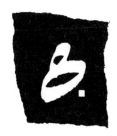

# Erotophobia
# Desire and Practice

"Erotophobia" may be defined as the terrifying, irrational reaction to the erotic which makes individuals and society vulnerable to psychological and social control in cultures where pleasure is strictly categorized and regulated. Each component of sexuality—sexual practice, desire, and sexual identity—constitutes a particular type of relationship between the individual and society, providing gripping opportunities for different forms of erotophobic repression.

Recent feminist and gay liberation theory suggests that gender and sexuality must be separated conceptually in order to understand, analyze, and develop strategies to cope with sexual oppression. The "sex radicals," as the new unorthodoxy has been dubbed, are heavily reliant on concepts developed by the new left, feminism, and gay liberation. Unlike the general tendency of the new left and orthodox feminism to relegate "correct" sexual expression to *after* the revolution (when women are free, sex will be liberated; when material relationships shift, sexual liberation will be achieved), the "sex radicals" argue that it is essential to understand the pattern and history of sexual repression *as a separate form of oppression*, not as one merely adjunct to or supportive of capitalist or patriarchal relationships. The impetus for this new thinking grew out of the sexual oppression experienced by some gay men, lesbians, and straight women within progressive politics. Feminism and marxism could not explain why sadomasochism was an exciting and revolutionary possibility for lesbians and gay men, why some straight women sought bisexual relationships that had more in common with gay than with traditional straight relationships, or why the right-wing backlash attacked areas of sexual freedom first.

It became apparent, though an embarrassment to some progressives, that the erotic is intransigent. The powerful physical longing that is contained within the imagery of sexuality spills outside the purely genital to eroticize a wide range of elements. Those who ventured into the theory and praxis of sex discovered that sex is more complex than imagined, and not simply determined by gender-role configurations. Desires are not easily controlled or categorized, but embedded in an unconscious grammar that creates feelings at odds with intellectual or political constructs.

Following the U.S. progressive tradition, the new unorthodoxy sought to create new theories of sexuality by describing a wide range of sexual experiences as they are felt today. The congruences and discontinuities between social and individual concepts of sexuality revealed patterns that provided clues to the construction of sexuality. The new theories relied heavily on the work of Jacques Lacan, Michel Foucault, and other European intellectuals, rendering much of the new theory difficult reading. Once sexuality was wrested from the domain of feminism, marxism, and traditional psychology it sat waiting for new analytical garb. There is scant language for discussing sexual experience that is not laden with the seedy if compelling language of the Gothic novel or the distastefully pristine terms of sexology. Ironically, the unorthodox bid for a language of sexuality that is closer to the physicality of desire takes an excruciatingly intellectual route. Still, there is fruit to this labor: the new models must ultimately be tested by their ability to analyze and generate strategies for the diverse personal and political struggles like AIDS, the sexual practice debates within feminism, and the re-emerging rightist trend toward penalizing all non-marital sexual expression with physical penalties of imprisonment, untreated disease, restricted access to abortion, birth control, and accurate information about sexuality.

The new models must be understood as methods of sorting out from a matrix of oppression components which in reality are overlapping. The most difficult element of this new project is its anti-utopianism, its refusal to reduce this oppression to one or a set of elements which, when eliminated, will leave a "correct" sexuality. The Foucaultian notion of discourse overlies or replaces the more traditional notions of primary causation or dialectics: the unorthodoxy looks for tears in an apparently seamless fabric rather than binary contradictions or root causes. This makes it difficult to feel wholly satisfied with new strategies: without a focal, linear history it is difficult to gauge progress. With sexuality, felt on an intimate, body-based level, each insight into one part of sexuality crashes into another inhibition or draws some new limit on experience. Each project, whether it is trying a new practice, or reshaping our sexual identity, seems less exciting or less congruent with desires than anticipated. Sexuality, as it is experienced today, unites the real and imaginary worlds, the lived practicality and the subjective experience. Much of contemporary Western sexuality exists in fantasy and daydreams, in longing and expectation. Because men's fantasies have been privileged over women's, and whites' over those of people of color, whole classes of people have been placed in danger. Feminists are suspicious, and rightly, of calls to unleash the power of fantasy: women have been victims of male-dominated sexual relationships too long. Nevertheless, fantasy and actual practice are separate and different: to view fantasy as the driving *sine qua non* of sexual practice leads to problematic strategies. Fantasy can retain qualities of ambiguity, impossibility, and a connection with atemporal desire that no experience at any given moment can have. By viewing fantasy as only one of many intrapsychic discourses that interact with social and cultural discourses operating by different sets of rules, the new analysis can observe the construction of the sexual subject in her or his *total* context. Creating and evolving fantasy can be a survival strategy for existing in a repressive society, particularly for people concerned about acquiring AIDS through sexual practice, and for others experiencing sexual terrorism as a result of the ideological backlash associated with AIDS. Understanding this new unorthodox feminist theory of sexuality and its possible contribution to resisting AIDS-related oppression requires a theoretical detour through the sex debate.

## The sex debates

The current "sex debates" spring from several other dialogues within a range of political movements, each of which is strongly influenced by feminism's decade-long analysis of gender and gender roles. With the exception of debates about gay males, the arguments that led to the sex wars discussed female sexuality more than male sexuality. Even in the discussions of gay male sexuality, feminist analysis and "feminine" ideals were embraced as useful in understanding the nature of being gay. The primary location of the discussions that led to the current heated debate was the feminist movement, although gay theoreticians and feminists within the left also brought the notions of gender and sexuality to the interstices of these movements. That the sex wars would create coalitions across movement lines, rather than perpetuating the conflicts between them, was hinted at in the wide popularity of Gayle Rubin's 1978 "Traffic in Women: Notes on the Political Economy of Sex," still widely cited by feminist leftists and gay theoreticians. As a barometer of change and continuity between the often separate feminist, left, and gay movements, it is Gayle Rubin's 1982 essay "Thinking Sex: Notes for a Radical Political Theory of Sex," among other contributions to the now notorious Barnard conference of the same year, that marks the coherent emergence of a sexual unorthodoxy.

Although it seems almost trite by now to rehash the significance of the ideas presented at the 1982 Feminist and the Scholar Conference at Barnard, some important battlelines were drawn there.[1] The "sex radicals," or unorthodox feminists, consolidated a new type of feminist theory that differed from the orthodox in several important respects. The term unorthodox is more accurate than "sex radical": although the theoretical battle is currently being fought out over sexuality, it has other important implications. One of the critical features of the unorthodoxy is its reassertion of the body as the site of human subjectivity, as the locus of the variety of features that shape identification with a particular race, class, gender, etc. Strategically, it is this body which holds the most promise for interrupting the seamless articulation of ideas that perpetuate oppression.

The divergence of the unorthodox wing, as it emerged in the Barnard conference and aftermath, relates directly to the lived experience of feminist activists and theoreticians. Feminists who had begun to explore the possible range of sexual expression had been led into some terrifying areas of the "female psyche"—places that had no names and, if spoken of at all, were considered by orthodox standards to be remnants of the patriarchy, the self-oppression of women. Yet, some of these women came back from the abyss of sex with exciting stories to tell: somehow, what had appeared as politically incorrect had been fun, transformative, empowering. Sadomasochism and the re-emergence of "post-feminist" butch/femme sexual practices among lesbians drew the greatest fire, and when certain of the women associated with this new exploration were invited (in their academic robes) to attend the Barnard Feminist and Scholar Conference, Women Against Pornography (WAP) activists in New York planned a zap action against the conference. It was a dim hour for "sisterhood" when WAP members leafletted the conference registrants—who had not yet had the opportunity to get a schedule and list of workshops—with pamphlets identifying particular women scholars by name as part of a conspiracy attempting to promote sexual perversion in the name of feminism.[2]

It became clear that the many sides in this debate could not always directly engage each other, because of fundamental differences in rhetoric, theory, and praxis. The assumption that women should "speak out" about their experience, and that experience would be fairly considered as part of the data for an evolving feminist theory, met a closed door when the topic was sexuality. Although the debate has been characterized as pro- and anti-sex, or anti-pornography and anti-antipornography, these classifications represent only single moments of the much broader clash between two very different views of the nature and meaning of women's experience.

The real anger and pain for feminists in this discussion of sexuality lies in the contradiction between two interconnected forms of oppression experienced by women: sexual danger—the areas where men have abused women—and sexual pleasure—those areas that have been shut off for most women, the possibilities that are just beyond reach if women are to stay in their gender role as good girls.

This new unorthodoxy shifted the terms of debate toward understanding sexual pleasure and the creation of subjectivity as both an enlightening theoretical innovation *and* a possible contribution to empowering women to combat sexual danger. Although there is a tendency either to see the two debates as separate or to view the discussion of pleasure as less important, it is undeniable that the unorthodoxy introduces new terms, realigns the relationships between old terms, and employs a different analytical method.

## Roots of a new theory

As feminists in the last few years developed new ideas about sexuality, the lesbian and gay movement was confronted with AIDS. The old tools of analysis were not sharp enough to make clear distinctions in a rapidly changing medical and political assault on sex. Although unorthodox feminists had new systems to offer, they were busy defending themselves against sisters who claimed they were brainwashed, reactionary, or unable to accept their self-oppression and change.[3] The marxian theories that viewed sexuality as channeled into work by capitalism may have suggested reasons why homosexuality was not widely accepted, but they also rested on the idea that sexuality runs wild until restrained by some force, perhaps by AIDS. Even gay liberation ideology was equivocal: if an initial goal was the assertion of "gay is good," then perhaps the solution to AIDS was to consider the years of promiscuity and exploration to be the community's "adolescence," which now (though admittedly tragically) should "mature" into "responsible," directed, even monogamous sexual expression. If the feminist, marxist, and gay liberationist perspectives left much to be desired in their ability to answer urgent questions, each was ripe with possibilities.

The post-structuralist philosophers offered the most useful tools for understanding the sex wars and AIDS sex panic. The essential ideas which marked the emergence of French structuralism as a critical development of both marxism and existentialism remain in the post-structuralist ideologies. Most important is the shift in questions and methods which emerged in particular with Foucault and Lacan, the most often cited and criticized of the post-structuralists.

Fascinated with language as a model for other areas of socialization, Claude Levi-Strauss, the most controversial and enduring of the structuralists, sought to understand "how the myths think themselves out in men."[4] Levi-Strauss' poetic insights into the relationship of people and their thoughts developed in later thinkers into a notion that language, and other practices, create subjectivity. A second important structuralist contribution to what would become a heated discourse on sexuality is the notion that materialist history and cultural study are really two approaches to the same problem; their methods differ, but both seek to understand human nature and change. Both are necessary to the project: the diachronic approach of history and the synchronic analysis of culture together project a truer picture of the forces and mechanisms that create human subjectivity, and the possibilities for changing consciousness.

Foucault elaborated his method by dancing through the various traditional academic disciplines: philosophy, history, anthropology. He used particular cultural concepts (punishment, madness, order, sexuality) and showed how various knowledge systems (science, economics, law) worked together through different periods of time to create the prevailing notions. He focused on the shift from the Classical Age to the Age of Reason, and often erected historical landmarks at places not generally expected. Levi-Strauss tried to apply diachronic and synchronic methods by delineating for each a proper domain. Foucault proposed a more coordinated method that linked these separate *discourses* with rules and patterns that interlace into a fabric of cultural consciousness. Although Foucault's followers use the notion of discourse in different ways, the shift in method is significant. It stands in marked contrast to the more usual historical materialist methods, and to the ahistorical and mythical methods of radical feminism.

Thus, where inheritors of Marx tend to view history as a diachronic sequence with important dialectical movements relating to material relations, which together give rise to ideology, inheritors of Foucault cast history (as it is linearly perceived), economic or technological
changes, and ideology into separate and more autonomous "histories"
or discourses. Instead of a dialectic which promises contradictions that
may be used to progressive advantage, inheritors of Foucault search for
the unasked questions or hidden discrepancies between coexistent discourses. Lacan's rereading of Freud provided additional guidance,
though his work is the most controversial of the "fathers" noted here.

    This differs from many feminist and gay liberation methodologies
because it does not refer to the consciousness-raising or "coming out"
events that form the experiential or pragmatic basis of both these
movements. While both may frame historical questions—who gained
consciousness throughout time and what structures prohibited this in
others?—and cultural questions—what systems must be built to support the new consciousness?—neither is successful at explaining how
subjectivity is created, and whether two claims to gay or feminist
identity are really the same.

    These new theories produce a new view of "gayness." While it had
been popular to view gay male oppression as related to women's
oppression because gay men act like or are socially classified as women,
gay male oppression is also related to the discourses that produce the
notion of *queerness*.[5] Women are also circumscribed by the discourse
on queerness, not only if they are lesbians, or even heterosexuals who
engage in particular types of sexual activity, but also when they suffer
the penalties of queerness by contracting AIDS. Although sexism,
racism, and homophobia all interlock to stigmatize people with AIDS,
and anyone perceived to be at risk, this stigma hinges most profoundly
on the discourses that elaborate queerness, or deviant sexuality. Erotophobia figures importantly as the operational mechanism uniting a
variety of discourses that have something to say about queerness.

    "Discourse," as used here, is a loose term referring to a discussion
or non-practical dialogue about an idea that is conceptually separate or
bounded. Ideas are interrelated, but the term discourse will be used to
refer to abstract groupings of interactions about an idea that is conceptually identified for the purposes of better understanding.

    Practices are an interaction that occurs on the practical level. They
refer to actual events or moments: making a film is a practice, having
sex is a practice. Practices are related to discourses, but in a less stringent or formal way than suggested in either marxian or radical feminist
theory. In marxian theory "praxis" is the embodiment of theory in the

real world. Orthodox feminism has generally assumed that people act out the ideology they have absorbed through socialization, and therefore has traditionally viewed practices as directly related to ideology. Following Foucault, practice is viewed here as the deployment of some part of a discourse. There are two operations (at least) by which this may happen. First, practice may be directly mapped from a discourse, as radical feminists have tended to suggest. However, practice may also relate to discourse through a series of transformations related to apparently separate discourses in a way that makes practice seem to contradict a discourse. Each practice must be carefully analyzed relative to many discourses.

Thus, as Foucault has argued, the Victorians had an extremely prolific discourse on sex, all of which sounded proscriptive of sexual practice. But historical documents suggest that Victorians may well have engaged in as much and as various sexual activity as earlier and later eras which are presumed to have been more "liberated." In the fabric of discourses that create the seamless culture around individuals, deployed practices may create ruptures or discontinuities so severe that the operations of the discourse can no longer account for them and the terms must change. Lesbian sex radicals claim their practice shattered the gender discourse that defines heterosexuality. Gay men, as will be seen, can create sexual practices that defy the AIDS-related rightist backlash and may shatter aspects of the discourse on queerness.

The question of subjectivity—how people identify themselves—and general epistemological questions—how people gain knowledge—are critical to political systems that analyze and create strategies to effect changes in consciousness. One of the major problems in orthodox U.S. feminist theory, which has been inherited by many gay theorists as well, is the very North American notion of "consciousness-raising," suspiciously derivative, if unconsciously, of the American pragmatist school of philosophy (Peirce, Dewey, Whitehead, James).[6] Some pragmatists tried to avoid the question of subjectivity by arguing that empirical tests of community standards reflect the values of the formed subject. The relationship of the individual and her/his chosen community becomes tautological unless there is a more complex explanation for the construction of the subject offered.

Consciousness-raising and pragmatism assume that by identifying those phenomena which make a difference in everyday life, individuals can agree on practical, moral principles which, taken together, form a community base. The concept of the "reasonable person" follows logically as the typical member of this consensual community. U.S. feminists were initially able to turn this homogenizing of common experience on its head in consciousness-raising groups (borrowed from the Black Power movement's method of "speaking out"). But, in the end, it was not a system that could incorporate the vast class, regional, religious, sexual, and racial differences of U.S. women. "Women's experience" was set against the presumptive "human," but actually male experience, creating a tacitly defined "reasonable woman." In gay consciousness-raising, the same summarizing phenomenon occurred, although the constant assertion of fringe sexual practices—forms of "queerness" based on violation of sexual taboos in addition to gender— lessened the normative power of "the average homosexual." This pragmatist method said little about what the various practical categories it discovered meant to different individuals.

The sex radicals offer a new approach to this problem by identifying in sexuality—sexual practice, sexual identity (or the articulation of subjectivity), and sexual desire (or the reading back onto the body of sexual identity)—conceptual categories that need different strategies if the individual and his/her community are to successfully cope with a problem like AIDS. Conceptual models reveal parallels and differences between sexual cultures which may promote or suppress different types of sexual practice, but separating elements and summarizing individual experiences into cultural trends must not substitute for speaking about the real feelings and activities of an individual. This form of empiricism, where the generalization is read back to the individual as the expected norm, is the very pragmatist trap this theoretical project attempts to escape.

The progressive discourse on sex is usually inarticulate and remote from individual experience. The most intelligent statements are couched in terms so far removed from how real people think about sex that they become meaningless. The discussions closest to people's lived experience are often charged with personal doubt or political inconsistencies. Sex manuals may explain "how to" but rarely express the excitement or terror of approaching the question "why." Polemics on sexual liberation by feminists, gays, or "fringe" sexual communities often inspire hope about positive sexual possibilities without explaining where to meet such fascinating people, or what to do with them once they are found. The presumption that sex is "natural" or "comes naturally" appears in right-wing diatribes against perversion and permissiveness as often as it occurs in progressive discussions of birth control, likes and dislikes, or fantasies that are suppressed because they make sex "too self-conscious." The body is left out of intellectual discourse as untidy, and intellectual ponderings are excluded from practice as "unsexy." The message right, left, and center seems to be do it, but don't talk about it too much. One purpose for the model of sexual practice, desire, and sexual identity, then, is reintegrating the mind and the body in a whole discourse that makes sex as exciting to do as it is to analyze.

## Gender

All societies build a multi-layered gender-role system: a meditation on perceptions of genital configuration in a social and economic context. In some societies, gender-role conformity is strictly enforced through physical sanction or ridicule, while in others, it is permitted to coexist with such widespread violations that the gender-role categories are functionally unimportant, but still imbued with ritual or religious significance. Some societies maintain rigid gender roles, but create a category for non-conforming individuals who are thought to have special healing powers—in essence creating a third gender not based on genital configuration. All of these methods serve to reinforce or even define gender roles, which then reinforce the notion of gender. But none of these methods conflates adherence to gender role with moral correctness quite as strictly as Anglo-American culture. In the absence of mythological or theological explanations for why women are expected to be one way and men another, biology and history vie for explanatory primacy, even in progressive politics. Men or women act a certain way because *it is natural*, either biologically ("they are made that way") or through careful analysis of their role throughout history ("see, they've always been that way"). To act another way is unnatural. Acting in disregard of the social prescription calls gender identity into question. Violators are not "real men" or "real women," but neither do they have the appropriate genital configuration to be a member of the opposite sex. They are cast into a half-light of gender non-conformity where the individual's experience of difference is still in relation to a world fundamentally divided by gender.

It seems obvious that there are two genders—male and female: this is one of the most unassailable perceptions in the Western world. The division of gender is based on centuries of Western myths, which contemporary U.S. citizens believe are supported by scientific data: visible genital configuration, the wealth of biological and pseudo-biological genetic and hormonal discoveries, argue that there are two natural genders. The appearance of disjunct data—Klinefelter's syndrome, hermaphroditism, gender dysphoria—is not taken as a sign that biology may be the least significant thing about cultural concepts of gender. Scientific anomalies reinforce the primacy of biology: these are the exceptions that prove the rule, biological accidents that reinforce the idea that genital configuration in and of itself propels the whole gender-role system. Studies have examined the relationship of adults' perceptions of a child's gender and the child's assumption of gender-role behavior, but these studies get hopelessly mired in yet other exceptions. Some children who are raised in contradiction to some biologically determined fact (special knowledge that the scientist has of the child's gender based on the hypothesis of hormonal or genetic determination), grow up to defy their socialization and assume the role of the gender they (according to scientists) "really are." Gender dysphoria—people who, though scientists may be unable to find any "rational" explanation (i.e., no genetic or hormonal anomaly, or, barring that, no aberrant socialization) experience themselves as being trapped in the body of the wrong gender—raises even more complicated questions about the significance of the biological basis of gender. Instead of re-evaluating the premise that gender is most importantly biologically based, scientists seek ever more refined methods for linking genital configuration with hormones or genetics or with some clever pre-cognitive impression of like and non-like.

Genital configuration plays a large role in identity formation, but for symbolic, and not for "natural" reasons. Reformulating the notion of how gender is constructed reverses the formula which now places biology at the root: gender construction is a symbolic process by which the individual—through a complex interplay of social, religious, psychological, economic, erotic, class, and racial factors—forms an identity. This model reduces the importance of gender *per se* as an organizing principle in the individual's matrix of identities, and introduces the idea that biological "facts" may be behavioralized in many different ways depending on the other factors of identity formation. Thus, gender is constructed at the socio-psychological level and read back to the individual who believes that it *feels* a certain way to be male or female, and that these feelings are "natural."

This form of empiricism is particularly acute in the United States, where the pragmatist world view insists on the primacy of the individual's perception of experience, a mask for the tyranny of the mainstream sensibility. Those who do not *feel* or experience their world according to the dominant cultural notions have their feelings translated for them through a prism which says, "You would feel that way if you weren't black, female, poor, etc." In the social change movements of the last two decades, disenfranchised groups have challenged this insistence on translating experience into the reality of the white, middle-class, male mainstream. But the "speaking out" of consciousness-raising created a new empirical model which then allowed for the notion of "more conscious than thou," which varies little from the original pragmatist model. Within radical circles, a shift toward constructionist notions of identity will meet with resistance from the neo-pragmatist model of understanding experience.

The notion of destroying gender by promoting androgyny that was so compelling to feminists and gay liberationists in the late 1960s, has in less than a decade given way to a mystical belief in women's superior nature and men's inherent sexual drive. Gentle men reinforce this new version of gender roles by trying to relearn the "feminine" nurturing qualities, which, by a perverse calculus, solidifies the bad "male" category of dominance and violence by being the exception that proves the rule. The binary calculus for identity formation continually projects two morally charged categories. When the categories are threatened it is easy to change their definition (it can be "in" to be a feminist man) but rarely is the basis of the categories challenged. There is an insistence that the raw perception of self has some innate qualities that precede the individual's entry into culture. But both the individual and the categories invent each other and constantly modify each other according to rules which are both systematic and contradictory.

## Practice

The idea of sexual practice moves away from a deterministic model based on biology. Once gender construction is stripped away from the construction of the sexual subject, it is apparent that either gender may practice activities that appear similar, even though the meaning and pleasure perceived by the two may be different. The different perceptions relate to social, psychological, and gender configuration, but the symbolic meanings may cross.

Talking about sexual practice allows for a clearer discussion of what an individual likes than fuzzy terms like "sex" or "sex acts"— terms that conflate what people do with how they or society feels about it. If there can be any objective discussion of sexuality, it is of sexual practices. Sexual practice is the practical strategy for uniting sexual identity and sexual desire, for uniting the individual's experience of sexual agency with her/his physical and psychological longings.

There are great differences in the articulation of sexual culture for lesbians, gay men, straight women and men. The notion of sexual practice is most strongly articulated in the gay male community in part because the male/male sexual practices destroy the calculus of gender configuration-determined sexuality, but also because in the U.S. men are socialized to feel sexual agency. Only a minority of urban gay men participate in the most elaborate aspects of this sexual culture, but the *idea* that many possible sexual practices are available has a major impact on how identity, practice, and desire coincide for gay men. The notion of broad sexual possibilities, together with a less absolute correspondence between sexual desire and identity, has positive implications for the possibility of changing sexual practice to align with "safe sex" guidelines.

## Desire

Desire—sexual desire—is perhaps the most hotly contested territory in contemporary Western discourse. Law, psychology, political movements on the left and right, all seek to define desire for their own purposes: to control the definition of desire is to obtain the power necessary to effect sexual liberation or maintain oppression. It is tempting, of course, to review anthropological literature and conclude that sexual desire is a universal human component, even if its representation and expression vary widely. This type of argument has been popular among feminists and gay liberationists as a hint at the possibilities of sexual liberation. Leftists often use these data to avoid dealing with human variation, presuming that such vast individual differences still add up to societies determined by a material base. These empirical formats for wrestling with desire are products of Victorian psychology, and represent but one of many possible ways of framing what are essentially epistemological questions about the body. While acknowledging the valuable insights of both psychology and anthropology, with their critical inquiries into the nature of modern questions about humans, sexual liberationists must look past the frameworks offered by these disciplines, which are typical of the rational sciences. Whatever other insights these disciplines or their radical political offspring may offer, they are nonetheless settled on the notion that desires are somehow inchoate, surging forces which are channeled or repressed in the practical world.

Although Lacanians view their theories as reframing this problem, Foucault argues that because for them desire is produced by the structures governing desire, they still accept the inescapable struggle between desire and power. Although Lacanian theories may have this limitation, they also suggest some practical applications that are difficult to draw out of Foucaultian analysis. Indeed, many have considered Foucault to be anti-political. In one of his last interviews, he argued in favor of pursuing change without political programs "if it does not mean without proper reflection about what is going on, or without very careful attention to what is possible." But this leaves activists with more clues about what to avoid than what to pursue. Lacanian analyses imply that change can occur through disrupting the discourses on their own terms. Semioticians working within cinema have moved in the direction of understanding desire as based in pleasure (as does Foucault) and of viewing desire as constructed through the processes suggested by Lacanian analysis.[7] Recognizing that these types of analyses are at some junctures contradictory, but also pose interesting strategic possibilities, begins an eclectic journey which questions the inherited understanding of desire, and suggests possibilities for reformulating the concept of what is without a doubt a profoundly felt element in the individual's sexuality.

The perception (and perhaps the experience) of desire as a powerful, barely containable force was consolidated as a concept by nineteenth-century psychology, most notably by Freud. Literature and science alike depict the modern experience of sexual desire as rooted in conflict—with other people, social structures, with intrapsychic perceptions of self-control. On the face of things, it can hardly matter whether Freud invented desire or whether there is a real base for it in hormones or socialization, since most will agree to experiences similar enough to be called sexual desire, whether located in the mind or the body. But this "desire" is a concept specific to post-Freudian U.S. culture, more concerned with the question of where desire is located than with how sexuality is related to subjectivity.

The structuralists argue that humans enter culture through language. Lacan makes much of the process of gender identification through the entry into a languaged world: language marks the body with zones and meanings. The body—the site of subjectivity—is created and en-gendered by language. Foucault takes this idea in a slightly different direction by arguing that sexuality and sex are created by the partitioning off of particular parts of the body, which are then identified as sexual. The particular parts and their assigned meanings shift for discernible historical reasons; nonetheless, the cultural category of the sexual remains arbitrarily defined. The individual's experience of sexual zones must be related to the matrix of race, class, and idiosyncratic elements, not simply reread through gender. Classically, for example, a shoe fetish is mapped back onto gender by identifying the foot as the phallus, the shoe as a cunt, or more simply by assuming the narrow-toed, high-heeled shoe as a personal symbol of female or the heavy, leather boot as male. However, taking pleasure seriously as an independent category that strongly influences sexual identity suggests that sexual practices can be reformulated to respond to crises like AIDS and still remain gay and sex-positive. Pleasures are sensual perceptions or interactions which when assigned to categories begin to create zones on the body. When pleasures and their corresponding body zones are given social meaning and value, there emerges a self-consciousness about the body. Subjectivity is not simply an awareness of the body as having senses, but a perception that those senses and pleasures carry a social evaluation. The recognition of these body zones with their attendant pleasures, and the evaluation of these zones and pleasures, invite the choice to pursue particular acts that will recognize the zones and pleasures. Sexual practice, then, is very early associated with pleasures—is accepted by the subject as the method of attaining particular pleasures. The subject's possibility of willing creates a sense of agency—a sense of being able to unite pleasures and acts in a system consonant with the subject's organization of the zones. But, of course, all zones are not equal, and they are arbitrary to begin with. Thus, from the onset, the subject's agency is potentially at odds with the available range of social roles. Although the idea of sexual pleasure may be universal in some form, the permissible acts for attaining that pleasure, as well as the exact content and extent of the zones designated as sexual, are still governed by laws of language, and supported by religious and legal mechanisms.

Desire is culturally constructed out of these categorizing projects: a meditation on pleasure and subjectivity. In any given social and historical period, pleasures are capriciously designated and correlated with body zones. Subjectivity is constructed by the possibility of agency in directing those pleasures. This is not the pleasure principle—the pursuit of pleasure and avoidance of pain—for the very categories of experience identified as pleasure or pain have undergone extensive definition before they are projected as possible outcomes of practice. Foucault argues that the laws and structures that deny pleasure or desire create that desire. But he does not mean that people exist in a sort of negative supply-side economy of sex where they only want what they cannot have.

Rather, he suggests that the attempts to understand sexuality empirically (deciding what sexuality *is*) obscure what pleasures are possible.[8] Thus, desire is a fraudulent conflation of pleasure and subjectivity invented in an era which sought to control sexual libertinism by attributing unconscious motives to sexual agency. Once sexuality, through the invention of sexual desire, is relocated in the unconscious rather than in pleasure zones, it becomes possible to invent perverts

whose sexual practice is symptomatic of misshapen subjectivity. Before
the invention of perversion by the nineteenth-century sexologists, sexual practice had to be controlled directly through law, family constraints, or moral dicta against particular acts. Although some socially
constructed zones were defined as illegal and some pleasures went
unacknowledged in the zoning process, the pleasures themselves were
not penalizable unless observed in an illegal sex act. This idea that
hidden desires drive the search for pleasure short circuits agency by
implying that a set of randomly assigned zones have absolute values.
Thus, for example, anal pleasure becomes absolutely identified with an
infantile stage of sexual development, which, if not outgrown, leads to
a certain course of subjectivity formation. The cultural consolidation
of this idea (first codified by Freud) in the early twentieth century
helped create the contemporary idea of sexual identity.

# Identity and Community

Erotophobia directs itself at one or more aspects of sexual practice, desire, or identity. As cultural concepts of gender, practice, desire, perversion, etc. fail to answer the normative and structural questions that organize sexuality, new concepts arise. "Sexual identity" is the most recent of the concepts that organize individual and social discourses about sexuality. Claiming a sexual identity in opposition to mainstream mores provides an escape for individuals repressed or persecuted for their homosexuality. Openly acknowledging the positive importance of homosexuality informs and integrates other aspects of the individual, rather than viewing "deviance" as a correctable anomaly in an otherwise normal person. Identity as a new mechanism for wresting sexual difference from the clutches of the erotophobic ordering structure that penalizes practice and desire enables a protective community to form new mores and a culture that supports homosexual practice and desire. Reclaiming the definition of homosexuality in a public community context made "gay" and "lesbian" positive terms in a whole identity that catalyzed the broader challenge to cultural concepts of difference that marked the early years of post-Stonewall organizing.

Greater openness and tolerance, and a stronger emphasis on sexuality as part of the integrated identity, cost the camouflage early homosexuals often had—despite greater individual struggles—and created a *community* which could become the target of erotophobic and homophobic strategies. Once "the closet" was defined, the individual had to be "in" or "out": homosexuality had now to be expressed in sexual terms *per se*, not refracted through ethical, literary, or artistic community. The formation of identity as a central principle of the emerging lesbian and gay community made it possible to deploy erotophobia in a genocidal form: rather than attacking or terrorizing a loose collection of individuals with a perverted component which they might hide or forfeit, a whole culture of homosexuality could now be destroyed. Individuals would now feel personally attacked if any aspect of their community came under assault. AIDS represents a unique assault on the newly emerging sexual identity and community in the U.S.

## Homosexuality versus "gay identity"

Various societies throughout history have articulated homosexuality and even homosexual roles. Ancient Greece, for example, celebrated male homosexual love, and homosexual practice flourished. But both homosexual desire and practice were conceptualized within a pedagogical context: gender and parental structures based on gender not only remained intact, but controlled the forms of sexual practice. A sexualized relationship between males was encouraged between students and teachers, but not among adult peers—except in some cases in the military where homosexuality served to further increase the male identification of early Greek culture.[1]

Many have argued that the great witch-burnings in the seventeenth century were a genocidal act against lesbians and gay men.[2] Some evidence supports the thesis that these witches may indeed have been homosexuals; however, the genocide was directed at *heresy*: homosexuality was a symptom of heresy, not the cause. Certainly, sexual practice was under assault, and perhaps even precursor communities, but it is difficult to argue that lesbian and gay identity as such was under attack.

In Western cultures at the time of industrialization, boys were permitted both sexual desire and practice with their male peers, although this practice was to be "grown out of" by late adolescence and desire was transformed into nationalism. The transition from adolescent sexuality to rigid heterosexual adult sexuality was pronounced for males, but often expressed in cultural symbols not directly related to sex. Male homoeroticism is observed in dramatic ways in the postindustrial era. For example, Nazi Germany's art is astonishingly homoerotic and served as a mechanism for integrating homosexual desires and anxieties into a nationalist identity.[3]

Until quite recently, notions of sexuality were profoundly based on gender, by either scientific or naturalist paradigms. Analysis of gender identity and gender-role compliance seemed to explain every-thing about sexuality. The notion that the male penis is the active element in sexual practice obscures any historical record of what females might have been doing among themselves.[4] The absence of a penis in female homosexual activity made lesbian relationships seem silly, futile attempts at male sexuality. Female masturbation was often punished, but homosexual activities were ridiculed, if they were noticed at all. In the rare cases where female homosexuality is pun-ished, the crime lies more in imitating men than in offending nature.

The omnipresence of male social and cultural power makes it easier to direct male gender identity and anxiety about sexuality toward national goals, but also highlights the ostensibly inappropriate sexual practices as "anti-social."

Until the industrial revolution and the invention of psychology, kinship, religion, and law organized sexuality by regulating sexual acts. Although laws changed and liberalized over time, the basic unit of legal sexuality was the married couple. Laws described a hierarchy of legal and illegal acts and, within the marriage unit, what degrees of violence, satisfaction, frequency, and types of sex were permitted. But this legalistic approach to the acts of sex sought to cope with sexuality by regulating *how* sexual agency was enacted. The idea that a sexual identity might guide choice through a dynamic meditation on sexual practice, desire, and self in a broad social fabric was not yet possible. Heterosexual identity did not exist until gay/lesbian identity highligh-ted the notion of agency in choice of sexual object, gender, and later in types of sexual practice. Individuals have probably always felt attrac-tion to persons of one sex or the other (or both), but the penalties and rewards for socially correct choice were primarily legal. Until some notion of sexual agency emerged, there were no "homosexual people," only acts that took place with a person of the same gender: homosexual-ity could be a crime or a symptom of insanity, but not a state of being.[5]

With the increasing reliance on rationalism and the gradual replacement of religious regulation with medical regulation, discus-sion of non-marital sex proliferated. Since heterosexual intercourse seemed to be "natural," it was spoken of less and less, while medicine began to study sexual differences, delineating perversions from the merely illegal. (For example, extra-marital heterosexual sex was close enough to the "natural" form that while it remained illegal, it received very little study unless it involved payment; then it was a vice.) Homo-sexuality, childhood masturbation, and eventually women's sexuality became the subjects of study, as scientific medicine attempted to catego-rize sexuality. But it was still a little longer before gay people and sexologists recognized a category of homosexual people, and then only in response to the intractability of homosexual behavior. Once defined into a species rather than juridical category ("outlaws" as opposed to just being illegal) homosexual behavior became identified as comprised of certain acts and qualities, and thus a possible choice or self-discovery.

The urbanization which facilitated the industrialization of Western culture played a large role in both consolidating the idea of sexuality and in demarcating the three categories of practice, desire, and identity. Until the industrial revolution, Western sexuality had been acted out relative to kinship and family networks. Cultural taboos, which were codified in civil and canon law, detailed whom one could and couldn't marry (the only legal form of sexuality). Rural areas limited the contact an individual might have with both possible spouses and possible illegal sex partners. They also created an environment where it was much easier to oversee individual behavior.

The industrial revolution brought together many young, single, unrelated people in an anonymous environment. Less subject to traditional forms of sexual regulation and enmeshed in a dramatic shift, many new urbanites could write their own rules. No solid examples existed for the factory worker, although many dormitories provided education and socialization into an urban environment. Historical records show that small friendship networks of homosexuals lived in many urban areas, quietly creating a subculture.[6] These early lesbian/gay communities were more like libertine societies than the lesbian/gay ghettos of today, often creating clubs of non-sex-related interests in which to express their homosexuality. The eighteenth-century libertines suggest a tradition of experimentation with different forms of sexual practice, but their overt role was usually protest against labeling some acts illegal. Because of the class privilege of most of those involved in these movements, such experimentation was identified as decadent—a hedonistic, vestigial element of a decaying social order. The emerging middle class, especially in the U.S., identified sexual license with the European regal establishment. De Sade was sweeping in his criticism of bourgeois and Christian sexual mores, coming closest to the contemporary separation between gender, sexual practice, and social organization, but his use of the pornographic political novel seemed horrid and evil. His political attack on bourgeois sexual mores is often missed because he is inappropriately read through Freudian lenses, despite the fact that his work appeared before sexology arose as a medical specialty.[7]

Boswell and others use the virtually universal existence of homosexual activity or laws against it to argue for a continuous history of
homosexual culture. D'Emilio, Weeks, and Bronski, in particular, take
a different view, arguing that homosexuals have existed throughout
history, but that a new and significant change occurred during and
after the industrial revolution. Each argues that the use of the term
"homosexual" must be period-specific, and claims that although there
are psychological reasons why contemporary gays and lesbians may
wish to find predecessors throughout history—or even identify a continuous, strict history of gays and lesbians *per se*—the radical shifts in
consciousness surrounding the secularization of medicine, the speciali-
zation of the bourgeois homosexual, and the emerging concepts of the
individual and community in the industrializing West make the direct
link with early consciousness of homosexuality impossible. All identify
a continuous process after the industrial revolution, even while each
proposes a different model. D'Emilio sees the formation of a homosexual community in the critical massing of gays and lesbians in urban
areas; Weeks sees the medicalization of homosexuality as predominant,
or at least integrally related to class shifts in the bourgeois; and Bronski
links class and scientific changes with the emerging culture of men who
relate their sexuality through their cultural interests, but assert an overt
"sensibility" of sex and pleasure. Each views the development of a
public sexual identification as a key stage in the process of identity and
community formation.[8]

New urbanites may have been introduced into homosexual friendship networks with subcultural codes but many found lovers of the
same sex through single sex rooming or work situations and were
engaged in homosexual activity before they fully realized that this was
not considered "natural." Indeed, court cases in England show that for
members of both sexes (but probably more often for women, whose
sexual practices were completely mystified—Queen Victoria is said to
have outlawed only male homosexuality because she did not believe
women engaged in any similar activity) brought to trial for "crimes
against nature," one party often had no idea that what they were doing
was a minority practice.[9] "Sexual desire," in the absence of constant
family supervision, could easily find a variety of practices.

Because there was less need to marry and adjust sexual desire to the
prescriptions of marital sex, the various sub-categories of activity
within homosexual (and presumably heterosexual) practice could
flourish and find more experimenters. Although assuming gender-role
behaviors seems to have been prevalent, it is not clear what relationship
gender identity had to sexual practice.[10] Certainly, there was not yet a

sophisticated critique of gender—homosexuality was widely considered a "third" sex, a biological mistake where gender traits were
confused in a person, or a developmental mistake, where the individual
was incorrectly socialized.

This very insistence—often by the gay people themselves—that
homosexuals had somehow veered off the course of heterosexuality
further confuses the meaning and political value of gender roles. Often,
only one partner in a pair was considered a true homosexual (butch
women, fem men) and the other was considered weak-willed, confused, indiscriminate, but essentially normal. The medicalization of
deviance created the seed for both sexual identity and for a profound
critique of gender, which would be elucidated, not surprisingly, by
feminist women and feminist gay men. Finally stating that individuals
*were* homosexual, and not merely that they engaged in homosexual
acts, created the condition in which individuals could contemplate
their sexual desires and the objects and operations of their practice. The
formation of identity subjected homosexuals to attack for mere *appearance*, but also created the possibility of rapid community formation
around new "gay" values. With the invention of the homosexual came
the invention of the heterosexual, the necessary opposite that is the
privileged category. But heterosexual identity did not develop in the
same way: the assumption that heterosexuality is *normal*, and that
heterosexual intercourse is "natural," allows desire and practice to
continue to be conflated for most heterosexual people.

## How cum they all live in San Francisco, or World War II and the creation of the gay ghettos.

The most important shift for contemporary Western lesbians and gay
men occurred during World War II, when gender separation intensified: women moved into traditionally male jobs and roles, and count-
less lesbians and gay men relocated in urban industrial centers to be
inducted into military service or work in military-related industries.
The U.S. case has been most clearly documented, but British and
German research, as well as anecdotal evidence from other Western
European countries, suggests that the intensification of lesbian and gay
*community* identity was a broad phenomenon.[11] The similarity of gay
male cultural institutions and ideology throughout Europe and even in
the major urban centers of Japan and Hong Kong suggests that gay GIs
shared their emerging culture abroad, and learned from other nascent
gay male communities (and to some extent, from lesbian communities). They encountered different ways of socially buffering homosexu-

ality, and thus alternative ways of protecting themselves. The similarity of gay male communities (and to some extent lesbian) across the industrialized world seems to argue that industrialization, coupled with major wars that brought massive numbers of single people into urban centers, was a condition for the emergence of contemporary lesbian/gay communities.[12]

One important aspect of this community development that has not been well recognized is that huge numbers of working-class, rural, and middle-class, non-urban gays became part of the urban working class when they received dishonorable discharges during and after World War II, or just decided not to go back home after a taste of a new life. As in any mass migration, lack of connections, housing, transferable skills, and jobs in general tends to level classes for a period of time. Lesbian/gay community formation in the 1940s and 1950s mimics ethnic migrations to a large urban area. In addition, the "last hired, first fired" rule put many civilian lesbians and gay men out of work when the war was over and vets came back to their jobs. It is no great mystery why Los Angeles, San Francisco, New York, Boston, Chicago, Atlanta, the District of Columbia, and numerous other smaller industrial urban cities should have developed gay communities. Having sacrificed home, family, and even career to become part of a semipublic, urban gay life, many lesbians and gay men seem to have taken marginal jobs that allowed them to lead an openly lesbian/gay life without having to worry about being fired. Many middle-class and well-educated lesbians and gay men with broader employment options found lucrative or professional jobs, but others—fearing loss of jobs if their homosexuality was discovered—took low-paying jobs where "moral turpitude" was of less concern and which wouldn't represent a great loss anyway if they were fired. Fear of job loss continues to serve as a prior restraint curtailing some gay people from seeking rigorous career paths where time, personal relationships, and greater involvement in the lesbian/gay culture must be deferred during periods of the career, and where the hint or disclosure of homosexuality would not be tolerated and career sacrifices could be lost in the single moment of coming out.

In addition, with the codification of a sexual culture and fewer demands in terms of the children and spouses of the traditional family constellation,' some gay men were at last free to opt for leisure over labor, a choice which allowed for greater participation in sexual activities, social and political organizations—activities which fused the emerging sense of sexual identity with a group identity that would in the late 1960s liken itself to a class or ethnic group. Without the

traditional myths of winning bread for family and home, gay men
with enough money to pay the rent and buy food had the new possibility of buying entertainment, sex or sexual meetings (i.e., entrance into
bars or bathhouses), and, in a sense, buying community—since the net
effect of this new freedom was to create what Michael Bronski has called
the "pleasure class." Volunteer time, enthusiasm for community-
building, and the good feelings of stabilizing one's community
through self-created institutions sent gay men, and to some extent
lesbians (who have much different economic constraints), into the
creation of churches, physical and mental health clinics, recreation and
entertainment, and political organizations.

But until the 1970s, most meeting places for gay men and lesbians
were non-gay-owned, requiring some cooperation with forces that did
not share the emerging social and political values of these new urban
communities. Gay men and lesbians were at the financial and legal
mercy of straight, often syndicated crime-connected porno stores,
cinemas, and bars. The new choices were undercut by overpriced establishments with little concern for protecting the rights and identities of
patrons. Low-income lesbians and gay men paid a high financial cost,
and the more professional, highly paid lesbians/gay men ran an even
greater risk of losing their credibility, family, and career if they were
caught in a raid or entrapped. This created community tensions around
money and privilege, coming out and staying closeted. The well-to-do,
openly gay business or professional (usually) man is a very recent
phenomenon. As the 1960s moved toward the fateful June night of the
Stonewall rebellion, the most frequented and nascent institutions of
the lesbian/gay community were heavily trafficked by working-class,
student, or marginal lesbians/gay men, and much less by the stereotyped upscale white gay man—the mistaken image which continues to
pervade AIDS as a stereotype in the popular imagination.[13]

## Sexual identity

It is hard for anyone living in the U.S. in the 1980s to imagine that
sexual identity has not always been an issue. Although there are historical moments which come close to formulating an idea of sexual identity, conditions are missing. There have certainly been homosexual
practices and pleasures since the beginning of time. But even though
collections of homosexually inclined people formed societies or networks and identified among themselves a shared history of exclusion
from the heterosexual norm, the idea that one *is* a homosexual is very

recent. Gender roles and gender identity (what a man or woman *is*) were sufficient to explain sexuality until Anglo-American culture consolidated the idea of perversion born of unconscious desires—a notion that suggested that sexual practice might not follow directly from gender assignment. The idea of perversion reopened the question of pleasure zones and subjectivity.

This new discourse on identity had to take place in a cultural context before the various individual homosexuals could reintegrate pleasure and agency, before they could decide that they *were* gay. Twin cultural concepts, especially strongly articulated in the Victorian U.S., provided the final condition necessary to move the discourse on sexual pleasure to the level of creating the concept of sexual identity, which may hold some promise of reuniting pleasure and agency. The idea of the individual as part of a community shifted moral judgment away from capricious external authority and replaced it with a sense of "community standards" supposedly arrived at by some process of social consensus. The arguments about the nature of the individual and the entry of the individual into community date from the responses to the Cartesian splitting of the mind and body which located the ego (self) in the mind. The concern over the relationship between this newly emerged concept of the individual and the community was particularly acute in the Victorian U.S. The American pragmatist movement at the turn of the century, which was widely influential in the works of William James and John Dewey well into the middle of the century, sought to relate the individual and community in a democratic fashion consistent with the culturally held religious and political beliefs of the U.S.

The shift toward the scientific method expressed itself in the acceleration of scientific and medical knowledge, but it also held a fascination for the secular philosophers who commented on the "American experience" and widely influenced notions of education, community, and selfhood. By locating the source of proper behavior in common knowledge—the interaction between the individual and community—these philosophers began to articulate the contemporary notion of identity. The introduction of a bastardized version of Freudian psychology into popular culture through film and novels in the 1920s and 1930s added another dimension to the quest for identity within the plural U.S. community. The "unconscious" became an intellectual fad in the inter-war years, and U.S. citizens, suspicious of European experts while at the same time promoting the consolidation of their own professional classes, were especially obsessed with the notion of sexual repression. By the time Freud was known in the U.S., the progressive social purity movements had already heightened popular concern with sexual morals while trying to silence the discussion of sex. The consolidation of the notion of the individual at this time of concern with sexual immorality created the possibility of deriving a sense of sexual identity which could be conceptualized as a function of community and compared with "the average person."

The idea of a sexual identity emerged in response to several questions created by the gradual separation of gender from sexuality. If there are perverts driven by unconscious desires to seek certain sexual practices, they must eventually come to know themselves as perverts, as dissonant when compared to the average person. It is not only necessary to find a large concentration of homosexuals in urban areas, freed from the family by the industrial revolution, but they must also gain a sense of sexual individuality that is set over and against the norm of the average person. The idea of a new standard of average person could be created by these newly conscious homosexuals only through the creation of a new community based on a different set of laws governing the conduct of sexuality, as well as other relational behaviors—for sexual communities have always carried with them other regulations, often of an aesthetic or moral order, as in the cult of the dandy or in Socratic Greece where men bonded and sexualized their relationships in the context of the believed moral superiority of the male principle.[14]

The distinction between subculture and community is essential here: within the U.S. experience community is understood as an agreed-upon pursuit of a group of people which defines an order that can be understood in the embodiment of a hypothetical average person who intuitively knows the "community standard." Counter-culture is a concept of much later origin, arising out of sociologists' attempts to understand deviance and ordered groups of deviants in a way that casts the individual as existing in an insufficient cultural web, and therefore not really participating in community. The new left and hippie movements of the 1960s viewed themselves and their activities as counter-cultural in a revolutionary sense—as antagonists who reshaped the dominant culture through a living example of difference or alternatives. Although many in the lesbian/gay movement of the early 1970s viewed their political activity as counter-cultural, homosexuals already had begun to shape a community and a culture which functioned in and as a wry subtext of the mainstream culture. This community formed as the ideas of the individual and the community were worked out in the context of sexual identity. The concept of sexual identity could only arise in a group of people who created the possibilities for their sexual practice apart from the mainstream community. The

urban gay male community, and to a lesser extent the lesbian community, have unique attributes not necessarily found among homosexuals
living in rural areas or in small towns which have no autonomous
lesbian/gay community.
  Sexual identity, then, is the final part of this model of sexuality as
it is today. Sexual identity is a complex structure projected from social
and psychological elements: it is still profoundly influenced by gender
identity. Further, since the notion of identity arose in part to "explain"
gay liberation, identity is easily conflated with practice; the strong
association between homosexuality and anal sex has heightened the
cultural interest in anal sex for heterosexuals. Whereas heterosexual
anal sex may once have been just a kinky variation—or, before the
Victorian transformation, totally illegal because it did not lead to
procreation—once the notion of sexual identity arises *vis-a-vis* gay
men, then heterosexual anal sex provokes the question of possible
hidden homosexual identity. The practice of anal sex may become
symptomatic of hidden homosexuality only after the idea of gay identity promotes the assumption that anal sexual practice is an important
part of sexuality. Identity allows the culture to scare people out of
sexual expression by implying that the very sensibility of the person
engaging in a particular act can make that act "queer" even if done with
a person of the opposite gender. Bisexuality takes on an entirely new
dimension in the post-gay liberation era, beyond its association with
the sexual liberation of the 1960s. In the 1960s bisexuality was considered "more natural" and part of an attempt to break down possessive-
ness in relationships. The new, lesbian/gay-identified bisexuality
views the gender of the sexual partner as part of the sexual practice, not
as a support of the sexual identity. This small group of new sex radicals
often identifies the quality of their relationships as being more akin to
gay or lesbian relationships, even while their partner may be of the
opposite gender. This notion is only possible when gender is reduced to
the practical, and desire is organized around specific practices rather
than by gender configuration.

## The sexual is political

Erotophobia may be observed in the history of methods employed to
inhibit the integration of sexual desire, sexual practice, and sexual
identity in a way that facilitates human agency. It is inextricably linked
with economic and social structures, as well as the very language and
categories of a particular culture. Economic conditions can set the
conditions for the practice of sexuality and certainly influence the level

of discourse available. Many women in progressive movements, for instance, feel that to be able to talk about sexuality at all is a luxury, that food and shelter are more important issues. And yet, the control of women's sexuality under the most stark economic conditions is omnipresent, and often an equally felt oppression. Historically, the discourse on sexuality has privileged certain parts of the discussion. Medicalization of sexuality in the late 1800s left the naming of sexuality to elite scientists. But even earlier, upper-class decadence was culturally associated with sexual license, and the logocentrism of the discussion since has placed the most vocal tools of argument in the hands of those who had power over language. But the error of progressives has been to imagine that since empowered white males monopolize the discourse, no one else is concerned with sex. In the struggle to liberate the *discussion* of sexuality from the church and state, and then from medical science, and to point out the mechanisms of race, gender, and class operating in and through sex, sexual politics often fails to liberate the bodies who suffer under this matrix of oppression.

The denunciation of sexuality as an issue is symptomatic of the erotophobia still working within progressive politics: sexuality is diverted into either the discussion of practice (which makes it a "bedroom issue" apparently devoid of symbolic meaning) or desire (which tends to animalize or neuroticize sexuality and pass it off to the disciplines of biology or psychology). But people mediate their physical wants and enact them in the process of their sexual identity formation. Unless sexuality is examined as a system of discourses deployed historically and constructed idiosyncratically in the individual, sexual politics will come up with blanks when it analyzes the relationship between sexuality and social problems.

The repression of sexuality focuses on different elements of sexuality over time. But because some part of sexuality always goes unspoken, unnamed, the subjective sense of sexual agency will vary. The notion of sexual identity is very recent, consolidating in this country only with the advent of the gay liberation movement in the 1970s. The whole notion of "lifestyle," and especially sexual lifestyle, fuses sexual identity with the material accoutrements believed to support sexual practice. Sexual identity for women is practically an anti-identity, a form of nihilism that takes sexual desire and projects it into romanticism, which is a fetishization of the symbols of pair-bonding without the sexual practice. The irony of gay liberation politics is that once they confront the legal and social structures with a positive sexual identity the discussion of sexual practice is elided. It is a common experience of lesbians and gay men to find that their liberal friends, who support lesbian and gay rights, become uncomfortable when confronted with the realities of lesbian/gay sexual practice.

AIDS is one of the first major post-gay liberation events that has forced a cultural examination of sexual practice versus sexual identity. Because the idea of sexual identity is not yet fully culturally consolidated, many people do not understand why some men might feel an identity crisis when asked to modify their sexual practice for health reasons. Even in the most elaborate gay theory, the process of gay identity formation is ambiguously articulated, and the role of sexual practice in gay identity is equivocal.

## The culture of erotophobia

Erotophobia is experienced in a complex of fears and elisions. Sexuality is often controlled through terrorism—as syphilis was explicitly used in World War I, when sex educators invented what they called "syphilophobia" in order to curtail sexual practice [15]—or by silencing the discussion of sexuality. Foucault has made much of the idea of knowledge and power as reciprocal entities, arguing that the control and direction of knowledge are power. The very power to write large the cultural questions that organize the concepts of an era enables the dominant culture to provide certain kinds of answers. Sexuality, in particular, is the thing that one is supposed to know how to do without having gone through a formal process of acquiring knowledge. "Sexual knowledge" (or *Carnal Knowledge* in the movie) is considered to be acquired in the act. Ironically, in this most technocratic, education-oriented society, sex is the thing to which the least committed and most ill-informed educational efforts are directed.

Erica Jong describes the U.S. consumerist sensibility toward sex as "the zipless fuck": baby boomers were raised to seek sex, if they must seek it at all, in the most silent, undiscussed, unplanned context possible. To plan for sex or consider how one might wish to engage in it is cultural treason against the idea that sex is unspeakable. The contemporary U.S. experience of and attempt to subvert erotophobia can be described by three "axioms," each of which comes into play when the previous one fails to incite erotophobia.

## The domino theory of sexuality

Like the U.S. concept of saving the world from communism by fighting battles in the tiniest, most unlikely places, there is a domino theory of sexuality. Freud articulated an early form of this emerging Victorian theory in his *Civilization and Its Discontents*, but even such progressives on sex as Herbert Marcuse fell into the same trap of believing that both the repression and expression of sexuality had overwhelming effects. Sexual energy, this axiom holds, has the power to take over a person's entire life. Sexuality by its very nature is obsessive: artists channel it into creating cultural artifacts, politicians into creating political order. Under the logic of the domino theory of sexuality, one shouldn't even talk about sex because to talk about it will make people think about it, and thinking about it will make people want to do it. Eventually, all of civilization will come crashing down around copulating masses.

Most people, after an intense period of sexual exploration (or many such periods throughout their lives), discover that life gets boring if all they do is have sex. Sexual practice is often most exciting in the context of other social practices, such as work and participating in cultural production. After a while, even the most wildly sexual beings discover that they can hang from the ceiling by their feet and have their partner pelt them with tomatoes all weekend, and still dress for success or don the factory garb and be at work by 8:00 a.m. Monday morning. The domino theory becomes suspect.

## You are what you do

Like the nutrition campaigns of the 1960s, which showed people eating massive quantities of junk food and then turning into junk food, the "you are what you do" theory posits that whatever one does for sex will cause some outward manifestation. Media consumers are bombarded with the idea of the smelly, sweaty, drooling sex pervert, but this is just an extreme on the continuum from the idea that masturbation results in hairy palms. People who are deciding that they might be lesbian or gay scrutinize themselves for limp wrists, or a too-masculine walk. Everyone becomes afraid that people will correlate some outward manifestation with an acknowledged or feared internal sexual proclivity. An inadvertent admission of interest in the same sex or an interest in employing non-missionary positions might indicate that there is something wrong. Outward signs of difference might indicate an inward form of disorder. People become afraid of even discussing sex for fear that they will discover they are perverts. Havelock Ellis notes a case of this phenomenon in his 1936 *Studies in the Psychology of Sex.*

> A married lady who is a leader in the social purity movements and an enthusiast for sexual chastity, discovered through reading some pamphlets against solitary vice [as masturbation was then called] that she herself had been practicing masturbation

for years without knowing it. The profound anguish and hopeless despair of this woman in the face of what she believed to be the moral ruin of her whole life cannot well be described.

Finally, when people decide that they really do like whatever sexual practice they have come to by accident or careful thought, a third form of erotophobia emerges.

## Normal is what's normal for you

Like the Geritol commercials, many people come to feel that whatever they do is normal and whatever anyone else does is weird. One must have a certain amount of complacency about the legitimacy of one's sexual practice, so that heterosexual missionary position enthusiasts have garnered the most recognition for the normalcy of their act, but gay people may also feel that certain gay practices are normal (because they engage in them), but others are not. Gayle Rubin has formulated this in a much more systematic way as the "hierarchy of sexual deviance," where there exists an ever-shifting line between what falls within the normal and what is considered outside of it. This axiom, applied in the context of AIDS, surfaces in the feeling of many liberals that homosexuality *per se* is fine, but that promiscuous gay practice ought to be curtailed.

The culmination of all of these theories is the intensified search for signs and symptoms of irregular sexuality. AIDS taps into all of these cultural expressions of erotophobia, triggering legal, psychological, and moral recourses aimed at suppressing gay male practice, some forms of desire (replacing practice with emotional bonding), and lesbian/gay community.

# Safe Sex

Sexual practice, and to a great extent sexual identity, were both attacked early in the AIDS epidemic. "Fast lane" gay men were among the first to exhibit AIDS and these cases received extensive scientific and media documentation. Promiscuity and poppers, supposedly mainstays of the urban gay lifestyle, came under attack, followed quickly by the discovery of a correlation between AIDS and "anal passive" intercourse. Correlative epidemiologic studies continue to show a relationship between number of partners and AIDS, and once HTLV-III/LAV was discovered, it too correlated with number of partners and with receptive anal intercourse. But the significance of these findings was unclear. On one hand, it was obvious that more exposure to an agent increased the chance of becoming infected by it. On the other, no one could prove that HTLV-III/LAV was a sufficient agent to cause AIDS. Even among researchers who believed HTLV-III/LAV was the significant if not sufficient cause of AIDS, the models for how it worked were contradictory.

In the face of conflicting medical information and a right-wing backlash which insisted that homosexuality was the *sine qua non* for AIDS, the various AIDS groups rapidly developed what were at first called "safe sex" guidelines and later, "safer sex," "sensible sex," or simply risk-reduction guidelines. Developed mainly within the lesbian/gay community, although heavily reliant on information from the medical community, pamphlets began to appear even before any agent had been identified. The guidelines and the philosophies of the educational campaigns promoting them have been controversial, especially between regions. AIDS groups have evolved a style and approach in their brochures that reflect sex-positive, gay-positive values, and convey a sense of individual responsibility in the context of community self-determination.

Conveying "sensible sex" information has been obstructed by the cultural erotophobia, which conflates practice, desire, and identity. Despite the best intentions of AIDS activists, guidelines are often perceived as judgmental and limiting. Numerous men have experienced the sense that modifying or eliminating a central practice means they "are no longer gay." Sex is often perceived as the cement in the gay male community: gay men fear that if sexual ties are reduced or deemphasized the community as a whole will disintegrate. Without community institutions and support for sexual practice and political action, some men fear that the identity they struggled to create will be destroyed.

Each local community has tried in different ways to reinforce changes in sexual practice that offer alternatives for supporting gay identity, as well as to suggest new ways of cementing community. There has been wide suggestion—especially as the AIDS crisis proves more intransigent—to pursue more monogamous relationships, even justifying this pragmatic change by calling it a natural development and maturation of the "clone" generation. But this suggestion rests on incorrect assumptions about gay male lifestyles and "sensible sex" guidelines.

Despite wide media and even scientific reporting, epidemiologic studies show that it is not primarily number of sexual partners in and of itself that creates risk for contact with the virus, but rather the exchange of body fluids by direct routes. Thus, number of partners is significant to the extent that those practices involve an exchange of semen, blood, or possibly saliva directly into mucous membranes or fissures. Conversely, monogamy per se doesn't decrease the risk if one or more partner is virus-positive or transmits an unknown co-factor. An argument in favor of fewer anonymous contacts is that it is easier to discuss past sexual history and current decisions about sexual practices with a known partner. Two recent studies from San Francisco and Chicago, however, indicate that coupling does not necessarily produce more discussion or safer sexual practices.[1] These studies asked gay men why they had not changed a range of sexual practices, most of which the respondents agreed would decrease their risk of getting AIDS. In the San Francisco study, men in monogamous couples, in primary relationships with some sexual activity outside the relationship, and with no primary relationship but multiple partners, nearly all agreed that they hadn't implemented desired changes because they perceived their partner(s) to be unwilling to make that change. The second and third most common reasons were "I like it too much to stop" and "It just seems like what is expected"—a more diffuse articulation of the notion that certain practices, or a constellation of practices, are what makes someone gay. The Chicago study showed similar results: men are making an effort to change, but often continue in practices they view as unsafe because they like the activity or believe their partners want to pursue it.

Virtually all studies show that gay men are decreasing the number of sexual contacts across many practices, with much less attention to the relative risk of the particular activities. Long-time activist Bruce Voeller has said that gay men are giving up the least favorite sexual practice and the least favorite drug. The logic of reducing numbers without modifying practices involving the exchange of body fluids is counterproductive. Researchers often cite decreasing rectal gonorrhea rates among gay men in the last few years as evidence of positive changes. But gonorrhea rates are poor indicators of sexual practice, at least with respect to AIDS. Unlike gonorrhea, which gay men have been able to reduce in incidence through treatment, early screening, and health education, HTLV-III/LAV exposure is probably life-long in the individual and will remain a significant health risk to the community as long as it exists in the disease pool. Unless new technologies arise, once the virus integrates into DNA, it is not removable; once the virus enters a population it remains there for the life of all infected individuals. Drugs may ultimately limit or disable the virus(es)' activity, but researchers do not currently know how to "kill off" this type of virus. (This is also true of many other viruses—herpes family, for example.) The comparison with rectal gonorrhea rates is misleading, even if they indicate change in practices or increase visits to clinics, which may have positive side-effects for decreasing AIDS incidence. HTLV-III/LAV prevalence in a population only increases—even if men make significant reductions in number of contacts—as long as any of those contacts involve exchange of semen or blood.

The stereotypical focus on gay male promiscuity in the absence of thoughtful programs for changing risky exchange of body fluid has set AIDS education efforts behind and resulted in a loss of credibility in these sex education campaigns. The government has provided virtually no support for education, and no projects to test the efficacy of condoms or spermicides relative to an AIDS agent(s) have been funded. The research empire's inattention to these areas of work and the insistence on number of partners when all data point to a much more complex constellation of individual and group behavioral dynamics is little short of gross national negligence.

Merely decreasing number of partners without eliminating body fluid exchange through the still untested use of condoms, changes in particular practices, or the possible introduction of effective spermicidal agents will not limit the spread of the virus.[2] As seroprevalence increases, further cutting back must occur to lower the odds of contact through unsafe sex. A much better approach is to focus on type rather than frequency of activity. Studies and pilot programs ascertaining how adjunct factors like drug use, anonymous partners, multiple partners, couples affect the process of making sensible sex choices are essential in overall risk reduction. There must be much more education about negotiating sensible practices in a subculture not yet accustomed to this new idea.

An unfortunate side-effect of what has been perceived as an assault on promiscuity is that some gay men now feel tremendous hostility toward the gay liberation movement, the activist gay community, and even toward themselves for what they now perceive as an "anything goes" attitude in place of true liberation goals. But this is a self-blaming process which will be ultimately devastating for a community struggling for individual and cultural survival. It is essential that AIDS education incorporate positive notions about coming out with the new information about necessary changes in sexual practices. Studies of men who have successfully changed their sexual practice show that the most important factors influencing their decision have been positive feelings about being gay and the sense that they are able to make changes that will be effective, along with knowing and remembering images of someone who had AIDS.[3]

AIDS groups around the country have varying relationships with the other lesbian/gay organizations in their towns. Where the traditional lesbian/gay activists have not been very involved in AIDS organizing, there is often an ahistorical tendency by AIDS activists to see themselves as having done the first community organizing, or even existing in opposition to activism they perceive as promoting "AIDS behavior." This results in part from the checkered relations between traditional activists and "clones" in many cities. The early activist sentiment that "if you aren't part of the solution, you are part of the problem" did not fairly credit the difficulty and triumph of mainstream men and women in their simple struggle to be openly lesbian/gay, even if other aspects of their lifestyles conflicted with the goals of the coalitionists. In addition, some new activists are defensive about their past lack of political involvement, feeling that if only they had seen sooner what was happening, they might have made a bigger difference. The failure to create and communicate a visible heritage about the wide variety of lesbian and gay struggles sometimes results in AIDS organizing that does not realize or acknowledge the extent to which it builds on the previous work of gay men and lesbians in many areas of civil rights, health activism, and in shaping a diverse image of what it could mean to be lesbian or gay.

In general, most AIDS groups have taken pains to celebrate gay male sexuality while making suggestions about health precautions. A few of the more community-oriented gay male sex magazines have followed suit by offering safe sex information along with porno stories and pictures.[4] The unwillingness of the traditional gay male institutions oriented primarily around sex to change their values has had a direct and, so far, not entirely positive effect on men's ability to adjust their sexual practice and still feel good about being gay. Baths and bars with back rooms, in particular, have not been very receptive to holding educational forums, or even passing out pamphlets. Recently, some owners and managers have come to realize that sex and AIDS education will not necessarily "hurt business," but the prevailing sentiment among owners and many customers is that the visibility of AIDS organizations in bars and baths is depressing and discourages any— even "safe"—participation in sexual culture.

Activists who have favored bringing legal sanctions against bars and baths feel that these owners have been irresponsible in responding to the health crisis and are "making money on disease and death." On the other hand, the legal brief against closing the San Francisco baths presents convincing data that in the absence of other educational efforts, men who chose to attend the baths and engage in unsafe sexual practices would engage in equally unsafe practices somewhere else.[5] If the baths could become an educational vehicle, argued the brief, they might serve a better purpose by staying open. The issues surrounding legal interventions are extremely complex: activists must weigh the historical and social role of institutions in the development and support of individual and community against the tradition of civil and physical attacks on lesbians and gay men by the powers who would supervise the closure of baths and bars. It has been all too easy in the process of developing sensible sex guidelines to confuse the sexual norms one might like to see with those that are actually risk-reducing. Many activists do not see the destruction of institutions that support promiscuity and anonymous sex as a loss. However, a credible, liberationist, "sensible sex" program must include clear information and the widest, most creative range of choices for a highly diverse culture of gay male sexuality.

## Safe sex: authority and masculinity

Compounding (primarily straight) doctors' uncertainty about modes of transmission is their basic ignorance about contemporary gay male sexual practice, identity, and community. And yet, medical people are presumed to be the "authority" on which forms of sex might be "safe."

Even the notion of "safe sex" is new for many gay men, precisely because they are men raised in a culture that leaves responsibility for the "safety" of sex up to women. Women are more accustomed to making the difficult and multi-layered choices about the psychological and physical safety of sex. Cast in absolute terms of "safe" versus "unsafe" by male researchers and gay men unused to negotiating the sexual economy from the object side, the discussion has denied the personal difficulties gay men would encounter in learning about and enacting sensible sexual choices in a sex-negative culture. Certainly, gay men had become aware of sexual health issues before AIDS—especially relative to gonorrhea and hepatitis B—but this concern was not well integrated into the whole fabric of gay male sexual culture. The early discussion revolved around individual acts and an individual's decision-making process—not as an entire cultural reassessment of sexual institutions and community-determined shifts in codes and mores.

This individualistic approach implied that every man was in it for himself, an approach which impeded a more interactive process of group change. Only by exploring the changes and possibilities of a sexual culture that reinforces safe sex can sexual practice be more realistically placed in its actual context of identity and community. Only when sexual choice is reframed from "do" or "don't" to how one might enact low-risk sexual practices commensurate with physical pleasure and identity, can the possibilities of transforming sexual responsibility from a perceived limitation into an empowering aspect of sexual identity emerge. With AIDS, gay men have been forced to consider risk and to take responsibility for understanding and deciding the possible consequences of their sexual practice. Like "coming out," this is a complex process in which loss of current psychological and community structures must be weighed against the danger of this disease. The subjective sense of agency, of making responsible choices, must be highlighted *as part of* sexual identity and eroticized within sexual practice if sensible sex decisions are to become consistently applied life changes.

In addition, since the resulting changes in community are happening so rapidly, gay men who decide to change their sexual practice must reinvent community in accordance with their new decisions. Many men feel they are the only one making a change and have no place to turn for support or to find partners amenable to new sexual styles. Most AIDS organizations have instituted a wide range of therapy or support groups to deal with AIDS anxiety, but an even broader range of programs that promote building community around the new demands on gay male sexual practice and identity must begin. This is not as simple as closing the baths or forming jerk-off clubs, although the latter is a creative step in the right direction. Changes on both the sexual and non-sexual levels of gay community must begin to integrate the growing standard of sensible sex as a method of maintaining the community. Sensible sex will only be widely accepted when it serves to integrate gay men into a community they have participated in building. Neither sexual fascism nor sexual individualism will meet the need for both agency and community that promotes informed, self-affirming decisions.

The idea of talking with partners or friends about factors related to sexual choices (previous health history, sex history, as well as the fears and desires compressed and heightened by the ever-present AIDS conundrum) is anathema to the self-image of many gay men. In a sexual culture that idealized anonymity and promiscuity, that lauded sexual exploration of any kind, the skills and expectation of more pragmatic and vulnerable kinds of discussion are hard to acquire. Correctly or not, the gay male sexual economy is viewed as highly competitive: insisting on sensible sexual practices is often perceived as *de facto* limiting choice or inviting rejection.

The urban sexual lifestyle—perceived to involve much sex of every variety, drugs, and a general disregard for physical limits—has come under attack from within the lesbian/gay community, medical practitioners and researchers, and the straight community intent on blaming some gays but not the whole community. Like a Greek chorus, the varied voices chime, "If you'd just settle down and stop fucking everything that moves, AIDS would eventually be licked." Gay and straight psychologists liken the brief years of the clone revolution to an "adolescence" and encourage gay men to grow out of rampant sexuality into mature relationships. The subtext, and sometimes the explicit direction, of this advice has been to advocate monogamy, or at least sex within a small circle of friends. While these pristine solutions, directly out of the public health textbook, apparently make sense in the abstract, they bear little relationship to the complexity of gay male sexuality and sexual community. For one thing, they imply that intimate couples will talk more and have "safer sex," an assumption disproven by the studies discussed earlier. And the small circle of friends sounds like a suicide pact unless sensible sex itself is the objective of the club.

The new right, and some gay and straight progressives who advocate closing bathhouses, claim that the problem is with those gay men who just can't control themselves. Although few AIDS activists see restricting access to these traditional institutions as a positive choice, many view it as a last-ditch effort—in spite of the complications and implications of asking the state to regulate sexual behavior: if it saves some lives, they argue, it is worth it. Others view AIDS as a tragic occurrence which has highlighted negative aspects of gay male sexual openness that they believe should have been changed long ago. It is unfortunate that people had to die before gay men would make changes, they argue, but that is the reality. AIDS becomes a form of retribution, larger and more ominous than merely a strange new disease. This moral component seems to make the tragedy more palatable for some people: the randomness of the disease can be explained with guilty accusations. The logical extension of this sentiment is that if gay men had conducted themselves differently, AIDS would never have happened—an idea which is used to attack both gay liberation, for not being more specific about germs in its cry of "gay is good," and the bourgeois excesses believed to support the clone lifestyle, as if consumer culture had created some sort of dispositional weakness that left gay clones open to AIDS.

## The future of gay sex

AIDS means more than just holding off on some sex with some people for a little while, and this has not been palatably articulated within the lesbian and gay community. Although longtime gay health activists see the connections between education about AIDS and ignorance about STDs in general, the realization that the gay and lesbian community will be living with AIDS on some scale for decades or more has not hit home.

A new approach to understanding gay sexuality must view both the long- and short-term needs and effects of the AIDS crisis, as well as the historical mishandling of STDs across a wide range of sexualities. Most difficult, the lesbian and gay community as a political movement must come to grips with the evolving sexual identity of gay men coping with new restrictions and new possibilities for sexual expression. AIDS is transforming political identity as well as sexual identity, and a new lesbian and gay liberation ideology must evolve that is informed by innovative concepts that link class, race, gender, and sexuality as they have emerged in the comprehensive onslaught of the AIDS crisis. Lesbians and gay men are experiencing the most dramatic scapegoating as a community since Stonewall catalyzed the contemporary movement. It is difficult to discern radicals from conservatives, liberationists from assimilationists, in the middle of a crisis that necessitates working with rapidly right-shifting political and medical establishments. A redefinition of lesbian and gay politics must take place on both strategic and theoretical levels.

Lesbian/gay liberationists throughout the AIDS crisis have insisted that AIDS must not be viewed as proof that sexual exploration and the elaboration of sexual community were mistakes. Not only must lesbians and gay men not retreat into the closet, but they must maintain the vision of sexual liberation that defines the last fifteen years of lesbian and gay activism. But as friends, visible and closeted, continue to suffer from AIDS and die, that rallying cry is heard with less enthusiasm, repeated with less conviction. And yet, it is essential to maintain the vision of community in order to navigate the difficult waters of political backlash. The central messages of gay liberation can facilitate the transition to the new sense of community that must emerge as a result of the AIDS crisis, just as new notions of community evolved through Stonewall, Anita Bryant and the right-wing backlash, and through the "clone revolution."

Interestingly, several studies of the psychological impact of AIDS on gay men's ability to handle anxiety and make the necessary changes indicate a strong relationship between positive gay identity and ability to adapt.[6] Ironically, as AIDS pulls the identity carpet out from under gay men, those who feel most positive about their sexuality and are able to reach out to the individuals and institutions in their community may be the most successful at coping with the sudden shift in their reality— not just in changing sexual practice, but in evolving new community support systems that help make sense of sickness and death.

The paradoxical message about lesbians and gay men voiced by the straight society as well as gay liberation ideology is that gay men and lesbians are different because of sexuality: sexual objects are different even if many people are bisexual across their life experience, styles and range of sexual practice are different, and the identity and community constructed by lesbians and gay men have different value and support difference. Lesbians and gay men have chosen to celebrate sexuality rather than hide it. Even if they have not individually or as a group overcome erotophobia, the existence of the gay and lesbian community itself substantially subverts its influence. Pleasure is the assumption of lesbian and gay culture, not the denial of pleasure. When the voices of erotophobia speak from within, lesbians and gay men argue back, for erotophobia—in combination with race, class, gender, and other oppressions—has the power to disintegrate the community and identity that have been so hard to win. The new task is to re-invent sexuality and sexual community according to sensible sex realities and gay male identity needs.

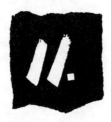

# AIDS Organizing

AIDS organizing is in many ways unique but dovetails with a long history of lesbian/gay and feminist organizing. Although AIDS organizing is the first activist experience for many of the gay men involved, most identify with the lesbian and gay community, a level of consciousness gained through the gay media, gay social networks, and the hard-won visibility of lesbians and gay men in mass media. Lesbian, bisexual, and straight women friends or lovers of gay or bisexual men have also become involved in AIDS organizing and also have an appreciation for gay male culture. The unarticulated "folk history" of the gay and lesbian community grounds the wide range of people involved in AIDS organizing within that community.

AIDS organizing brings the best of gay and lesbian organizing together with some of the movement's obstacles; the quality and direction of AIDS organizing promises to exert a major influence on the lesbian and gay community for years. Lesbian/gay health care will never be the same: the increase in awareness of sex-related health issues and the sense of empowerment about community control of sexuality and health, despite the tragic destruction of AIDS, will move sexually related health care problems to a more acknowledged status. The political lessons and networks established during the AIDS crisis will realign the political forces and the sense of entitlement of lesbian and gay activists who follow. The successes and failures of AIDS organizing will spin off other organizing efforts that will apply new or refined principles to other problems within the lesbian and gay community. A "post-AIDS" sensibility will emerge with a special emotional quality and political commitment, much as a "post-Stonewall" ethos resonates in lesbian and gay organizing after 1969.

The approach to organizing and community-building within the gay and lesbian movement after Stonewall had an enormous effect on the shape and attractiveness of AIDS organizing. Although many claim that AIDS "is not a gay issue"—and rightly—it is certainly an *organizing* effort indelibly marked with the concerns of a nascent community that validates non-biological relationships, promotes self-determination, and believes strongly in the dignity of the individual. The contemporary lesbian and gay movement experienced the peaks and valleys common to any political/cultural movement; however, to look mainly at the size of marches or the number of gay rights ordinances passed misses some of the most important aspects of community development that laid the foundation for a remarkable response to the many problems of AIDS.

The structural underpinnings of the lesbian and gay community that went into the AIDS crisis and the current trends in organizing around AIDS and other issues suggest the kind of community that will emerge. Because of possible new interactions between lesbian and gay organizing and traditional sources of structural power, AIDS will prove to be a major watershed of lesbian and gay organizing, whether tenured activists like it or not. Many saw AIDS as a diversion, a side path on the road of lesbian and gay liberation. Its size, duration, and the massive right-wing backlash it has engendered, however, mark the AIDS epoch as pivotal for the history of gay politics.

Gay and lesbian organizing has been forced to grapple with the diversity and isolation of gay men and lesbians in the U.S., and around the world. A major obstacle continues to be the historical invisibility of individual lesbians and gay men and their forms of social organization. Although the advent of industrialization and the massive demographic (and consciousness) shifts of World War I and II created conditions for the building of gay and lesbian communities in urban areas (Chapter 10 treats this in greater detail), the individuals who made up those communities were still more dissimilar than they were alike. The diversity of the gay and lesbian community has stimulated both creative organizing solutions and bitter divisions.

The tie that binds this community together is a shared history of oppression: the similarity of contemporary lesbian/gay communities in the industrialized West, a mark of the coherence and strength of homophobia and erotophobia, the nearly seamless fabric that encompasses bodily oppression through the nexus of disease and sex deployed to promote racism, sexism, classism, and heterosexism. Generally, the lesbian and gay community has tried to cope with the many differences through a celebration of the unusual, the camp and cultural, rather than through a unified theory of oppression. The result has been a mixed and painful ghetto where societal oppressions are still mirrored in the emerging culture. Many lesbians and gay men have chosen to identify with a community still marked by classic forms of prejudice rather than with their ties to class, regional, ethnic, or racial cultures which deny their sexuality. Other lesbians and gay men have stayed in their indigenous culture, and their accommodations provide other models for asserting a rich, complex identity.

Enormous cynicism and fractiousness exist among veteran gay and lesbian activists, as the apocalyptic promise of lesbian/gay liberation has failed to overcome racism, sexism, classism, and even homophobia within the movement. It is not surprising—or different from progressive movements whose members had more in common with each other from the outset—that the lesbian and gay community should appear at its strongest when reacting to overt attacks. The persistent ability to mobilize and fight back has been evident in AIDS organizing as about a dozen major AIDS organizations and several dozen smaller groups came into being almost overnight. AIDS organizing benefits from, and is in some cases hindered by, a series of trends and tensions that have been magnified in the post-Stonewall era, although some extend back into the very formation of gay and lesbian identity and community consciousness in the U.S.

## AIDS organizing

The emergence and progress of AIDS organizing around the country and as a national effort conformed fairly well to predictions based on local case incidence and previous history of political organizing. The same battles that had been fought within each community, and nationally, on other issues were recapitulated. The dramatic differences between east and west coast, and between the coastal areas and the midwestern and southern cities were rearticulated. The regional differences in sexual community, political organization, and general social acceptance of homosexuality created almost irreconcilable needs and strategies and hindered national organizing efforts. Yet, the National Gay Task Force, long in an unfocused state and out of touch with its constituency, was able to marshall its forces and what was left of its credibility to organize some national lobbying efforts. Their internal conflicts were much reported, and the vast diversity and historical differences between the various lesbian and gay communities and net-works in the U.S. prevented a comprehensive national program.

The mainstream and even alternative presses, as well as people in positions to help or ignore organizing efforts, believed that the lesbian and gay community was wracked by infighting, the perfect stereotypi-cal representation of the bitchy, backbiting queen. Allegations of infighting by outsiders are a common ploy to discredit grassroots efforts, and rarely examine the real and sophisticated differences a community is attempting to address. In reality, the lesbian and gay community's ability to act in concert, to employ its existing local and national organizations, and to continually tread the middle line between immediate action and long-term political commitment has been remarkably successful. In the AIDS years, many of the people in a position to move and shake were white men, often more privileged to "pass" than their brothers of color and their sisters, and often relatively unconnected—at least initially—with the longstanding lesbian/gay organizations. The relatively early and ongoing discussions of race, class, and gender differences reflected in AIDS created a possibility of challenging internal community prejudices as broad analysis and stra-tegizing evolve. Nearly every AIDS group has been forced to deal with the additional problems race, class, gender, and ethnicity create for people with AIDS. The interconnection of these forms of oppression is glaring to even the most neophyte activist. Still, AIDS organizations reflect the racial and sexual disparities of the larger lesbian and gay movement and mainstream U.S. society. AIDS organizing presents an opportunity to begin again, with a new understanding of these prob-lems within the lesbian and gay community.

AIDS organizing began at a time when many tenured activists were burned out, discouraged, cynical. The new recruits who carried the apocalyptic torch seemed hopelessly naive, and even seemed to be headed on courses that contradicted early lesbian/gay liberation work. "Clone politics" were growing, as mainstreamed lesbians and gays began participating openly in the electoral processes that traditional radicals could not stomach. It was Reaganland, and the liberationists were groping around for the light switch to end the nightmare.

The hard edge of experience with sell-out politicians and cor-rupted systemic power added an important dimension to AIDS organiz-ing, even if the number of old-guard radicals was extremely small. The new AIDS activists were optimistic and angry, often overestimating their ability to get assistance from the mainstream institutions. The war-weary radicals were on hand when the newly political came run-ning home with their tales of outrage and disbelief, producing a creative fusion of traditional lesbian/gay liberation politics with the new reminders of lesbian/gay oppression. AIDS confirmed the importance of and added new dimensions to the range of concerns treated by the previous decade of organizing. Although hard-line tenured activists have for years expressed exasperation with those whose only political activity was to read a gay newspaper or attend an occasional lesbian/-gay pride march, the values transmitted through these cultural exercises formed a subtle and tacit agreement about political concepts—the new activists were an educated but inactive reservoir. The "clones" who seem so visible in AIDS media coverage had been dismissed as apolitical materialists who gained a gay identity by acquisition of a look. While criticism of economic disparity is valid, clone culture did provide a positive, visible if material gay image, identity, and community that easily translated into political activism, even if the new activist style was less confrontational than in earlier years.

The danger of "coming out" through AIDS organizing is very real: even though there are many straight people involved in AIDS work, the grassroots workers and those working in the community are immediately suspected of being lesbian/gay. Straight doctors and nurses can be considered noble to work on this "gay" problem, but people who would actually become involved in the community are suspected of "going native." The involvement of straight friends has, however, created a new dialogue between admittedly small elements of the straight and lesbian/gay communities. The Boston AIDS Action Committee jokes about "heterophobia" workshops, but working closely with straight people has created new political demands. If political principles dictate that the people involved in community work should have some control over processes, then how do you deal with straight employees and volunteers in predominantly lesbian/gay organizations? In addition, lesbian and gay AIDS organizers deal with heterosexual people with AIDS and must offer sympathy and support to patients' families who have no other place to turn. From small things like the hostile remarks about "hets" from gay men and lesbians exacting a little revenge to the real political implications that lesbian and gay demands for acceptance must ultimately grant the right to a liberated *hetero*sexuality, theoretical and strategic discussions of the meaning of sexual liberation have been renewed by this dialogue.

## Disasters

The lesbian and gay community has been particularly susceptible to random "picking off," a form of terrorism that makes queerbashing or lynching of racial minorities a particularly effective deterrent to aboveground organizing. Bars frequented by lesbians and gay men have always been subjected to police raids where customers are beaten up by recreational pugilists who lie in wait for their gay prey. To many lesbian and gay organizers (particularly middle-class ones with greater access to private spaces, such as apartments) bars were bad for the lesbian/gay community because they encouraged alcoholism. Bars have promoted destructive individual patterns, but even in the largest cities entering a lesbian or gay bar is an act of self-declaration, and a necessary social focus for lesbians or gay men who have nowhere else to meet.

Bars and baths have been particularly subject to fires, a bizarre hazard wrought by the inadequacy of rundown facilities. Like the media image of black rioters in the 1960s who were portrayed as self-destructively burning their own ghettos, local media hype the angle that disgruntled customers or just crazy lesbian/gays have burned up their own spaces. Within the criminal justice system, lesbians/gays are labeled firebugs, vindictive and vicious people who attack their own community.

Persistent media images (including the controversial movie *Cruising*) make much of the supposedly "repressed" or self-hating gay man and his potential for destroying other gay men. Society is not blamed for driving gay men crazy, and lesbians and gay men, presumably programmed for self-destruction, are imagined to be doing each other in. The media coverage of disasters and murders within the gay community assumes that the perpetrators are "macho"-type gays, not nelly queens. The sexism and homophobia of this stereotype is pathetic: feminine men drive macho queers crazy so the machos knock off the nellys, who—since they are limp-wristed sots—can't defend themselves. And the macho gays would have just lived their lives as heterosexuals anyway if the nellys hadn't driven them nuts. The lesbian/gay community fights back against disasters perpetrated by negligence or active attack with a veritable "Red Cross" volunteer effort. When gay or lesbian churches, bars, or other establishments have been destroyed, furniture, food, money, clothing, and solace appear without even a request, with the donations coming from all segments of the community. There is a regenerative quality to lesbian and gay "institutions" that transcends the physical space. Amy Hoffman, speaking on behalf of Boston's *Gay Community News* after their 1982 fire—set by a ring of ex-firemen from Boston—summed up the ethos of community: "We still have ourselves."

Lesbians and gay men know that, like any marginal community, theirs is at the mercy of property-owners who would be happy to cash in their insurance policy at their expense. Yet, the image of self-destruction that is part of every U.S. lesbian and gay man's socialization makes each "victim" wonder whether one of "us" may have done it.

## Queerbashing

If disastrous fires leave a lingering doubt about members of the community, queerbashing raises a specter of another sort.

Since many queerbashed men and women fear loss of jobs or families if their homosexuality becomes known, they will not even report the violence against them. Lesbians and gay men who do report violence often experience ridicule and dismissal from the police. Queerbashing is a national pastime, the sort of youthful activity that makes real men (and future cops) out of unruly youth.

Much lesbian and gay organizing has revolved around protection from queerbashing. It is extremely unusual for queerbashers to be "brought to justice," and lesbians and gay men, often victims of judicial process, are ambivalent about sending queerbashers off to jail with the illusion that "justice has been done." Organizing around violence against lesbians and gay men has focused on self-defense through classes and awareness, solidarity through promoting willingness to risk defending or assisting a brother or sister even if it puts one in danger of exposure or ridicule, and through legal pressure. None of these activities has been lastingly effective, although each has been successful in stemming anti-gay/lesbian violence in certain settings for a period of time.

The difficulty of coping with queerbashing, although it has taught lesbian and gay activists ongoing lessons about dealing with homophobic assault, is that the victims are blamed for somehow placing themselves in jeopardy through their insistence on seeking sexual pleasure. (You wouldn't get beat up if you didn't go to the reeds for sex...) Like many other forms of attack, any given subgroup never imagines itself as vulnerable until it happens close to home: thus, it is some *other* type of lesbian or gay man who is assaulted. The experience of working together to prevent physical assault, and the desire to believe that it couldn't happen to oneself are dynamics carried into AIDS organizing.

One particularly interesting connection between issues surrounding AIDS and previous organizing around queerbashing is the issue of public sex. Several major community efforts in Boston (dating back to the earliest post-Stonewall organizing and running as a constant theme through the present) have focused on the Fenway, the primary outdoor cruising area for metropolitan Boston. One commentator links the attempts at solidarity in a response to queerbashing in the Fens with a revived interest in engaging in positive sexual activity that is lower on the risk scale.[1] He also notes that the type of anonymous, or semi-anonymous, sexual encounter that is the *sine qua non* of outdoor cruising is *promiscuous* by its nature, but may not involve practices high on the risk scale.

The whole topic of promiscuity has been a volatile one within lesbian/gay discourse. The usual lines between "radical" and "conservative" rapidly break down around the question of promiscuity. Before AIDS there was substantial discussion about promiscuity, with some extolling it as a mark of gay male sexual liberation, and others claiming it mimicked male privilege and duplicated the avoidance of intimacy associated with the macho ethos. Proponents of promiscuity remind critics that promiscuous gay men very often have a lifelong partner. The promiscuous aspect of their sexuality is another dimension, not a substitute for "real" sexual relationships—which, pro-promiscuity apologists claim, ape the constraining heterosexual relationships built on property and male domination that lesbian/gay and women's liberation criticize. The anti-promiscuity elements often see promiscuity as a futile expending of frenzied sexual energy, excusable as a reaction to years of repression by straight culture, but permissible only as a "stage" of gay male development. There are more important battles, they argue, than winning the right to fuck whenever, however, and wherever.

This debate within the gay and lesbian community has grown particularly intense in the AIDS crisis and in the recent upsurge of interest among some lesbian feminists in exploring a wider range of sexual possibilities. The "sex question" creates points of dissent, but also the possibility of renewing the commitment to radical notions of lesbian/gay liberation that have gotten lost or seem outdated as the movement as a whole has drifted toward civil rights and reformism.

Some of the problems of articulating the importance of lesbian and gay sex relate to public image, but others have major policy implications for AIDS organizers. Continued celebration of promiscuity in the face of AIDS—a disease blamed on too much fucking—seems to perpetuate the idea that homosexuals are essentially self-destructive.

## Dancing with the left

A major and important trend in gay and lesbian organizing in the past decade has been the attempt to form coalition with the left. Lesbian/gay liberation and the straight left have had a checkered history at best. The gains by progressive lesbians and gay men in finding a place in the "rainbow coalition" were in part won by submerging lesbian and gay issues. The emergence of AIDS created a crisis for lesbians and gay men involved in the progressive left coalition. On one hand, AIDS was somewhat embarrassing: political lesbians and gay men initially saw AIDS as a disease affecting the men who existed in the non-political social sphere. The real terror felt by lesbians and gay men as friends were lost and the entire community came under attack was difficult to communicate to straight comrades who had never been forced to deal overtly with gay male sexual practice. On the other hand, the funding and public service aspects of AIDS provided a concrete agenda item which progressive lesbians and gays could demand to have included on the coalition agenda. In the rush to expose funding and governmental neglect, the broader political and intensely personal aspects of AIDS— especially the effect on sexual culture and community—were substantially obscured.

It became hard to predict which way straight leftists might go when faced with questions like closing the baths. The idea of "saving them from themselves" observed in the right-wing response was also present in the concern expressed by the left, even if the sentiment was more sincere. By offering personal concern without strategic support, the left offered little assurance that they understood the importance of sexual community self-determination.

The discomfort that at least some lesbians and gay men have felt with the response of the left to AIDS is directly related to the historical relationship between the U.S. left and the gay/lesbian liberation movement. Despite support for lesbian/gay rights, straight leftist theorists have tended to add "gay" as a subcategory of sexual repression already understood to exist under capitalism. Feminist/leftist theorists have often been more supportive, although until recent theoretical work by Gayle Rubin, male homosexual oppression has usually been viewed as existing to the degree that gay men are like women (see Chapter 8).

On a practical level, whatever new left theories claimed, the realities of urban lesbian/gay liberation were considered a bourgeois distraction or a "lifestyle" politic.[2] When drag queens threw bricks at cops outside the Stonewall Inn in 1969, traditional leftists of all stripes spotted some revolutionary potential. After a few years of courting, the practical implications of lesbian/gay liberation ideology seem too hard to take. Marxist sectarians were willing to educate the new militant gay consciousness, but were unable to see the campy, confrontational style of early 1970s gay liberation as a legitimate form of politics. Lesbians and gay men within the left and leftists within the lesbian and gay movement have developed various analyses suggestive of a coherent theory, but neither the left nor the lesbian/gay liberation movement has made a substantial theoretical impact on the other. In the tentative coexistence of these political forces, lesbian/gay liberation—because it deals inescapably with sex—is usually the first oppression ushered out the coalition door when the ideological shit hits the strategic fan.

The cultural oppression of lesbians and gay men has not been understood by the left. Lesbians and gays are visibly oppressed to the straight left only when they are attacked in queerbashing, FBI harassment, or Anita Bryant or John Briggs-type campaigns. The more fundamental issue of homophobia—fear of homosexuals or homosexuality—rarely surfaces as a political idea worthy of analysis on its own. By consigning homosexuals to the list of people who must be tolerated despite some peculiar difference, the left does not offer radical gays anything more attractive than the mainstream political organs of the lesbian/gay rights movement. The general failure within the left—even where feminism has trod—to grasp the profound and anarchistic possibilities of liberating sexual identity from gender, class, race, renders much lesbian and gay liberation cultural critique and agit prop incomprehensible.

There is no good answer within the marxist/socialist tradition for how to strategize for sexual liberation, despite interesting work by Reich, Marcuse, and less systematic writers. Much of the "free love" of the 1960s was harshly criticized by feminist refugees from the macho new left. Homosexual praxis of the polymorphous sexuality thesis left lesbians and gay men feeling ripped off by straight comrades "slumming" in their fragile culture. Sex is among those things that will take care of themselves after the revolution: no one is sure how, and with that dim vision one scarcely knows how to conduct oneself now. Too much attention to sexuality is petit bourgeois, claim sectarians, baffled by the persistence of this topic. And besides, the workers are too busy for sex. The refusal to observe sexual cultures throughout all sectors of society robs marxists/socialists of the possibility of a much better economic and political analysis, to say nothing of a better comprehension of the ways in which ideology is created and reinforced in the intimate power dynamics of the sexual economy.

The inability to value sexual expression inverts marxist/socialist analysis of sexuality: the proliferation of sexual practice within the gay male community is viewed as an excess, rather than decrying the *lack* of free sexual expression within the heterosexual nuclear family (worker or not). Sex is rarely placed on a par with "material" needs, even though sexual practice and identity are profoundly interconnected with material relations. (Do they have private spaces for sex? Can they escape the close scrutiny of family and state? Can they get birth control? Afford admission to bars?) Despite ample excellent historical work by feminists and lesbian/gay historians that throughout industrial history "workers" have sought out and structured a sexual world, the left agenda-setters still duck the topic.[3]

It was no great surprise, then, that the left did not immediately leap up to volunteer for duty in the AIDS crisis, even though the people with AIDS included activist leftists, racial minorities, working-class people, women, prostitutes, and drug users. There were many obvious reasons which could have brought leftists or feminists into AIDS organizing that had nothing to do with supporting lesbian/gay liberation. It was the early and persistent misidentification of AIDS as a purely gay male concern that caused subtle and obvious blocks to a broad coalition effort to combat the most dramatic display of the failure of the medical empire in this century.

## The left and AIDS

There were several obvious points of juncture between left/liberal movements and AIDS organizing, all of them noted by the prominent journals, none of them followed up organizationally. Several sectarian or non-sectarian left groups organized panels or workshops but almost none took an active role in AIDS politics. The All People's Congress/-People's Anti-War Mobilization (*Worker's World*) is something of an exception, since they took a lead in covering third world issues in AIDS, including a panel on black gays and AIDS, and showed support for AIDS-related issues at lesbian and gay events beginning in 1982. However, no broad coalition effort has materialized, as neither the left pursues the AIDS issue nor do the primarily lesbian/gay AIDS organizations pursue leftist support.

The left has abandoned not only the lesbian and gay community, but also prostitutes and drug users—already seeing AIDS-related state harassment—and Haitians fought virtually alone to negotiate the international controversy about their inclusion in the risk groups. Many developing nations are experiencing AIDS with a strong implication that poverty and inadequate medical practice rather than sexuality provide the dominant character of the crisis. In one sense, it is appropriate and consistent with community self-determination that these groups have not offered a sexual prescription for the gay male community. However, as AIDS moves into the "straight community"—via IV drugs or queer sex—the left's uncomfortable silence about sexuality and AIDS leaves lesbian and gay activists wondering what the hidden sexual agenda is. As a portion of the left has developed a "pro-family" progressive agenda, with a renewed emphasis on future generations, the fate of sexual liberation is unclear. How long will the left provide even a modicum of support (which has really been more an absence of disapproval than direct political support) when AIDS cases increase and spill over into the straight population? Will leftists' latent homophobia mirror the new right's accusation that as long as gay sex goes unregulated, no one is safe? *Worker's World* and *Village Voice* both took stands against closing baths, arguing for community education and the right of each gay man to decide for himself the risk of going to the baths. Their tone stands in marked contrast to other liberal and left publications, where incredulity about the alleged number of sexual partners casts suspicion on gay men rather than on the quality of sexological research.

In the one-shot major AIDS articles in the *Nation, In These Times* and *Mother Jones* "isms" were all connected.[4] Gays are being scapegoated; they are experiencing from the health care system what women and poor people have always experienced (as if gay men had heretofore received good health care); funding priorities for AIDS research and health care are skewed; Haitians are being scapegoated for racist and anti-communist reasons (the allegation that AIDS started in deepest Africa, was transported to Cuba by mercenaries serving in Angola, then to Haiti where rich queers picked it up on their sexual vacations); maybe the CIA did it. Nowhere are the sexual partner numbers challenged, nowhere are the intricacies of medical research and FDA policies fully explored in relation to AIDS, nowhere is there a hint that science may *not* be able to solve all problems even with properly directed funding.

Everyone duly noted that sexuality was on trial, but few admitted which side they were on, or seemed to realize that their *own* sexual possibilities were jeopardized by the verdict. Gay men are in a whole different ballpark, these articles seemed to imply. Sexual liberation for gay men is different, their demands are greater (perhaps excessive); they want more partners and more positions, whereas *real* sexual liberation (for women and straight men) is about responsibility and equality.

To a lesbian and gay community used to random, terrorist attack, AIDS felt like genocide by an unknown force. Leftists did not grasp the implications of 5 to 10 percent of the gay men in each U.S. lesbian and gay community dying in the next few years, not to mention little understood neurological and other non-fatal complications for the some 40 to 60 percent of gay men exposed to the alleged virus. That half to a million people from highly stigmatized groups would face chronic illness, death, disability, poverty, uninsurability, and discrimination was dwarfed by the left's inability to resolve its ambivalent position on sex.

In addition to less than coherent analysis of lesbian/gay liberation issues and AIDS, the left has done little beyond lip service to analyze the situation of, or work for, Haitians, women, or IV drug users with AIDS. There has been little analysis of the experience of even the urban white gay male's experience of AIDS—for example, the effect of searching for public services outside the support network of the traditional family. The homophobia within the Haitian community and the racism within the lesbian/gay community continue, with both groups ostracizing their own members—the effect of germphobia. There has been no analysis of IV drug user cases—most left publications continue to call them drug *abusers* when they write about them at all—a strange twist of fate given the time and emergy put into drug law reforms in the 1960s and early 1970s. Discussion of prostitutes or any of the 800 U.S. women with AIDS is practically non-existent, and only *Worker's World* picked up the story of prisoners with AIDS, despite years of prison organizing by the left.

Other than discussing how AIDS has fanned the fires of homophobia, and to a lesser extent racism (in some accounts, particularly the otherwise good article in *Science for the People*, one gets the impression that before AIDS, the gay rights/liberation movement was not experiencing any new right backlash), there has been virtually no intelligent discussion of the broader implications of AIDS—the potential for the disease to jump boundaries, or even a criticism of the boundaries. Leftist accounts view each risk group as discrete and isolated; but bisexual males, recreational skin-drug users, and non-Haitian women (and men) involved with at-risk Haitian men provide several points of crossover. More immediately, left strategists have paid little attention to the reality that the political effects of AIDS *are* jumping boundaries. The legal precedents set concerning disclosure of health information, the refusal to include sexual activity under the

right to privacy laws, and the trend toward defining what complications of non-mainstream "lifestyles" will be covered by health insurance and discrimination statutes will certainly affect innumerable
future projects of straight leftists. Despite disclaimers within left coverage that AIDS is not a "gay plague," and criticism of mainstream
coverage, the left has failed to aid the reader or organizer in questioning
why research continues to look at only "gay" factors—promiscuity,
sexual behaviors.

Once the left journals' connect-the-dot analysis was complete,
readers were left with the illusion of a political analysis, and answers to
questions they did not ask. It still sounded like a gay plague. It is
difficult to explain in the age of AIDS why there must be a renewed
fight for lesbian/gay liberation without having straight friends wondering quietly whether this wasn't just a little like mass suicide. Whatever problems straight (especially male) leftists experienced about
sexuality, few faced the threat of violence or death for asserting the right
to their sexual practice. The medical and political AIDS crisis was an
extreme form of penalization for sex, different in degree but not in kind
to lesbians and gay men struggling for a positive identity. Sexual
freedom is less dear to the straight left because for heterosexuals sex is
substantially protected. Because heterosexism and erotophobia have
not found their way into the progressive coalition pantheon of Bad
Things, there is no consensus that they must be addressed. The incredulity of leftists at the insistence on sexual freedom is merely an intensification of the left's longstanding attitude toward the lesbian/gay sexual community: sex just isn't worth getting beaten up in an alley, swept
up in a bar raid, or possible getting a life-threatening disease over.

## An AIDS agenda

A broad agenda for AIDS organizing must be welded together by the
many kinds of people affected. People with AIDS and related illnesses,
as well as those in at-risk groups and those who will be affected in the
future by the medical and social policies set during the AIDS crisis,
must all recognize their common interests.

The cues for organizing will come from those who have been most
actively involved to this point—gay men and some straight and lesbian
supporters, Haitian activists, and IV drug community members and
organizers. Other social change movements have declined to become
involved to date, and although they must act quickly to come to terms
with the implications of AIDS for themselves, they must also accom-

modate to an agenda already in formation. Those who have not yet
become involved—directly or adjunctively—must first understand the
history, nature, and problems of the various communities most harshly
affected—including the poverty-related AIDS in the third world and
some areas of the U.S. Only with this understanding can their valuable
experience with other types of organizing be effectively incorporated
into AIDS work.

Ultimately, a broad AIDS agenda will include restructuring the
delivery of health care, more community involvement in development
of research priorities, reframing social concepts of sexuality, and identifying progressive ways of understanding difference that promote
human and cultural integrity. Although this seems like a large task, the
history of recent lesbian and gay organizing, with its attempts to find
commonality with other progressive movements, provides a solid
foundation for coping with these issues.

AIDS is not a "gay" disease, but it is a wide social problem for
which lesbians and gay men in the organized U.S. movement may be
uniquely suited as leaders. The U.S. lesbian and gay movement has
reconstructed its history and asserted its culture by fusing traditional
civil rights and legal activism with the anarchic contradictory style of
agit prop designed to subvert social restrictions. The respect for and
celebration of the idiosyncratic, autonomous person in the context of a
community which must negotiate vast differences in order to pursue a
common agenda provides a rich personal community experience of
viscerally felt politics—which holds important lessons for many other
progressive movements.

# Epilogue

I had tremendous difficulty being "done with" this book. I thought somehow that writing a work of such length would explain AIDS...most of all to myself. But there are no neat conclusions, at least not in 1985, for the problems raised here, and each of us must continue to grapple with finding meaning in the lives and deaths so sharply drawn around us. The contradictions lived and the understanding abstracted must complement each other or either component will strangle us. The personal and political lessons learned at such a great cost must not be lost.

Moments of clarity and of contradiction stand out in my mind. I had hoped to find a way to draw them more directly into the text, in some way to describe the texture of experience that informed the broader vision I was grappling to create.

One of my earliest memories of contradiction comes from a large meeting—it must have been the fall of 1983—when I first met Kevin. He and Bob got into an argument about how to deal with hospital staff who were insensitive about AIDS. Bob said he wanted to chase the doctors and nurses down the hall and bite them, screaming "I'm going to give you AIDS." Kevin grew angry and said that a quieter approach was in order, that we couldn't jeopardize the relationship for all patients in order to get angry in one instance.

Kevin was later diagnosed with AIDS. His sense of *doing* for the community, working in a way that benefited everyone, continued, although his militance increased. He was no longer one for quiet solutions. He stopped coming to meetings after a certain point because it became difficult for him and for the rest of us to keep his anger in proportion. He was confrontational, but it was too easy to write him off as a special case or to patronize him. He wanted us to fight back— against the problems he encountered and fight back with him, when he was off the wall. But the imminence of death made it difficult, and I, at least, erred in the direction of treading too lightly. Kevin was always a fighter. Like so many people with AIDS, he would talk about "beating AIDS," but when he said it, there was not the sense that he personally would be the one to survive. He would say, "*We* are going to beat it, someday." His spirit gives me the conviction to go on when it would be very easy to feel each death as another failure. Kevin, as demanding as he could be, saw the life of the community going on, creating meaning for everyone, even when the life of an individual ceased.

Moments flashed past when I realized how naive, how limited my own experience with death, and with life. Time and again, people working more directly with the people with AIDS would say that they had met and become friends with people they would never have encountered otherwise. Words are inadequate to express the powerful smashing of personal and groups borders that occurs in AIDS: death and the struggle to make a foreshortened life worth living level many prejudices and cast us on a trajectory to quickly identify the essential value of human life and personal interaction. The intimate experiences of AIDS organizing, the little successes and failures, make the big picture seem a little more manageable. Yet, at the same time, the dignity and hope and despair that are part and parcel of the direct care of people with AIDS are often overlooked in the bitter fights over funding and fair treatment, against prejudice and ignorance. The homophobia, racism, and sexism so grandly displayed in AIDS are also part of the daily experience of people with AIDS. They add insult to injury for the people whose stark reality is life and death, tremendous need, and bureaucracies that fail to meet them at every turn. I learned the most important lesson about the interconnection of many struggles from a person I will call Anna.

I met her on one of those days when I encountered the gamut of AIDS issues. I retyped a part of this manuscript that morning, adjusting edited parts, adding and deleting as the spirit moved me. Very abstract, moving words around, transferring ideas about AIDS to clean sheets of paper, which at some point would form this book. Sitting in my own little room I could say anything, be as confident as I wanted that I had the answers.

In the afternoon, I went off to interview one of the major AIDS researchers. I had usually gone to these interviews with *GCN* newswriter Chris Guilfoy, and I felt inadequate to deal with this interview alone. I had a hard time following some of the researcher's answers, and I didn't really get what I wanted from the interview.

Afterwards, I went to visit Bob—our friendship had solidified around AIDS organizing. In the time in Boston before there was a standing AIDS group, we argued and analyzed and generally got the reputation of being hysterical. We grieved over the deaths of friends and got angry at people we knew who still dismissed the AIDS crisis. On this day, Bob and I talked for an hour about how little had changed in the AIDS picture since we had co-authored an early article on the lesbian and gay male community and AIDS; how easy it was to let work, financial, and political obligations make us too busy to see friends; how some of those friends were now dead. We made another promise—never really fulfilled—to live more for the present. Bob asked if I wanted to visit Anna. It was so simple. It would be my first visit to someone in the hospital with AIDS.

I knew Anna was a transsexual; I did not know she was Puerto Rican. My next forty minutes would be a painful course in the construction of the prostitutes' community—the bond of ethnicity that transcends other differences—but most of all, I learned that dignity is possible, and a bitter battle to win. Even in the face of prejudice, death, and the sterile environment of the hospital room, Anna demanded it. I sat and listened. I didn't know what to say, and felt I had nothing to offer. She and Bob discussed her medical situation, she explained her current hospitalization to me. She described thrush and how it felt, her previous hospitalization for PCP. She was weak and concerned about paralysis. She couldn't lift the thin, cotton blanket into a warmer position. Bob and I gently moved it and tucked her in, careful not to hurt her sensitive, frail body.

"It's so heavy," she said, as we covered her six-foot, once husky body. We had to switch off the TV remote control, because Anna no longer had the strength to control the buttons. "Usually I just press until it lands on the right channel which turns it off," she said. "Sometimes it takes a while."

Shortly, her husband called. He had started going to AA at her request. She proudly describes raising his two children, and tricking the social service agents who tried to take them away. Her best friend—a prostitute—also calls. Anna explains to her what she wants brought from home. Her friend says she was hassled the last time she came in. "Just tell them you're my cousin," says Anna. "You're 'Rican, too, and they think I have a million relatives." She laughs as best she can. "And

honey, please bring my pretty pearl earrings. I look so ugly and I'm
tired of them calling me 'sir.'"

I wanted to cry. I could not fathom the amount of torture Anna had
faced—even before she got AIDS. An exception among exceptions, but
with such strong friendships. She tells about working through her
AIDS diagnosis with her family and friends, helping them overcome
their fear and anger. She complains about her best friend's new boy-
friend, and tells me that she hopes to get out of the hospital soon
because one of her boys wets the bed if she is away.

I remember an earlier moment, going to the Gay Men's Health
Crisis circus benefit. Thousands of people enjoying the camp and
fantasy of the circus in the midst of death and terror. There was such a
feeling of wanting to *do* something, if only we could figure out what. It
still seemed short-term. I was sitting near Arthur Bell, who died not
long after of a chronic illness. Even in the age of AIDS, old age and
other illness take their toll, although they receive less notice.

At this year's lesbian and gay pride march, I see the lover of a man I
know who has just died. The lover, a very quiet man, is walking
silently, in tears, carrying the placard bearing the date of his lover's
death.

One of the staffers from the AIDS Action Committee looks tired
and I ask her what's wrong. "We were up late last night," she says. "We
had to add two new placards from yesterday." The signs seem macabre
to many people, I know, but no one can think of another way to bring
home and commemorate these deaths.

At the top of the hill in front of the State House, we begin a chant
asking for the governor to restore the AIDS funding. In the middle, a
gay male leftist friend—whose lover died of AIDS last year—and I look
at each other.

"I never thought I'd be asking for government money," he says.
"Me either."
"But it's too big," he says. "We can't do it ourselves."

The next day, I see about two dozen of the new volunteers at
another rally against the governor, this time about removing foster
children from lesbians and gay men. Some of them are new to politics
and are overwhelmed by all the connections. Others, I realize, have been
there all along. I learn that one of the men I met through volunteer
work has just been diagnosed with AIDS.

I remember visiting a man I had met when he was very sick. He was
so thin and frail that he could only wear soft warm-up suits and had to
move with a walker and sit on special cushions. He was incontinent,
and wore diapers. He was too weak to talk for more than half an hour or

so, but wanted urgently to tell his story in some sort of coherent context. He had been a brilliant young physician, and was to have started pursuing clinical research. I remember taking notes for him. He talked so slowly, barely following a train of thought. I would look up above his head and see the beautiful, large prints of pictures of him taken by his lover only a year or two before. The face had aged a thousand years, but the lines were the same. I had to keep reminding myself that he was in his early thirties, just a few years older than I. When he went into the hospital—for what turned out to be the last time—I was afraid to visit. I knew that he might not remember me (he had often forgotten our appointments) and that he barely knew me at that. I wished I had met him sooner, had been able to be a friend for longer. I wish that I had known how to go to visit him when words and conversation were no longer possible.

One day, in my busy, often frantic state, I ran into one of the men with AIDS who had worked closely with me in organizing a conference. I said hello and immediately launched into my problems. Midway through, I stopped, speechless. He said, "You think you shouldn't complain to me because I'm going to die, don't you?" I mumbled my way out of a direct positive reply. "That's okay," he said. "I still have all of those dumb problems too, and they're real. It is nice to know everyone is still having the same fights and the same job stuff."

And life does go on; sometimes it just turns out to be shorter than we expect it. A lot of priorities—daily and political—have shifted, and not always very easily. I was constantly torn between taking on another committee obligation and putting in time working on this book. I started it because a very close friend, who I had drifted apart from, died when I did not even know he was sick, and because another man with AIDS, who died soon after, helped me believe that there were important things to say. I have finished it not out of some romantic wish to repay the deaths, even though I realized, as I completed this epilogue, that some of the people to whom this book is dedicated would not live to see it in print. I finished it because my experiences with people with AIDS and AIDS organizing renewed my faith that we can beat this thing, in all of its political, medical, and personal dimensions. We may not accomplish this in any of our lifetimes, but the process will enable us and our community to survive.

# Notes

## CHAPTER 1

[1]Dallas Doctors Against AIDS was the first widely visible group to use AIDS as part of a concerted anti-gay campaign. Dr. Paul Cameron is considered by rightists to be an expert on homosexuality. A more extensive discussion of right-wing ideology and AIDS appears in Chapter 7.

[2]Stereotypes about lesbians and gay men are ambiguous and change over time. The primary theme in homophobic stereotyping is that homosexuals are abnormal or unnatural, but this "deviation" may be due to too great a dose of gender traits (operationally defined as gender *role* conformity) or too small a dose. Thus, gay men may be hyper-male, and therefore promiscuous, or overly feminine. Likewise, lesbians may be hyper-feminine, and therefore afraid to go near men, or overly masculine.

[3]Bronski details the relationship between U.S. mass media and gay male identity in *Culture Clash* (Boston: South End Press, 1984).

[4]See Carol Vance, *American Psychologist*, November 1984.

[5]Eric Rofes, "The Revolution of the Clones: an Interview With John Preston," *Gay Community News*, 27 March 1982.

[6]See Barbara Ehrenreich, *Hearts of Men* (Garden City: Doubleday, 1984).

[7]William Ryan, *Blaming the Victim* (New York: Vintage, 1971).

[8]See Eric Rofes, *I Thought People Like That Killed Themselves* (San Francisco: Grey Fox Press, 1982).

[9]As this book goes to press, actor Rock Hudson's AIDS diagnosis made international news. This was the first major case of a public figure getting AIDS. In every conceivable media source covering the story, from the *New York Times* to the *National Enquirer*, the "tragedy" was as often AIDS as it was Rock's unmasked homosexuality. The

implications that Hudson was seduced into his lifetime of homosexuality does nothing to increase sympathy toward the gay community imagined to have caused his "fall," and thus, his illness.

## CHAPTER 2

[1]The following information on Legionnaire's disease is taken from Gerald Astor, *The Disease Detectives* (New York: Plume, 1982), pp. 17-40.

[2]This figure was cited by New England Red Cross officials reporting on the success of volunteer donor deferral at the Public Responsibility in Medicine and Research (PRM&RC) conference on the legal and ethical aspects of AIDS, 24-25 April 1985. Unlike media reports over the summer of 1985, which credited the HTLV-III anti-body testing with the decrease in post-transfusion AIDS cases, New England Red Cross officials viewed educational programs within the risk groups as largely successful. Most of the HTLV-III positive units implicated in transfusion-related AIDS cases were drawn before the major donor education campaigns in 1983.

[3]Michael Callen, a person with AIDS active in New York AIDS organizing, has challenged the idea that people with AIDS were "previously healthy." He argues, correctly, that many gay men had chronic and repeat infections of various sexually transmitted diseases. The medical industry's general disregard for overall sexual health and the broad cultural view that STDs are the price paid for sex allow this disease history to be considered "previously healthy." Medical professionals have made a good case for this distinction—the previous infections were not life-threatening and the gay men were generally in sound health.

[4]Preliminary results of a prospective study conducted by the Centers for Disease Control (CDC). See the *Morbidity and Mortality Weekly Report* (MMWR), 6 April 1984, pp. 181-182 and an update by Dr. Eugene McCray at the International Conference on AIDS (ICA) in Atlanta, "Prospective Evaluation of Health Care Workers with Prenteral or Mucous Membrane Exposure to Blood from Patients with Acquired Immunodifficiency Syndrome."

[5]Brandt discussed this decision in "Health Policy Implications of AIDS," an address delivered at the International Conference on AIDS in Atlanta, 1985.

## CHAPTER 3

[1]New York *Native*, 27 August-9 September 1984.

[2]*New York Times*, 24 April 1984.

[3]*Wall Street Journal*, 6 July 1984.

[4]New York *Native*, 18 June-1 July 1984.

[5]As many as 150 variations on the virus have been identified, but it is not known whether the differences have any practical significance. Dr. Martin S. Hirsch, a researcher at Massachusetts General Hospital, reviewed the implications of these findings in "Prospects for Therapy for AIDS Virus Infections."

[6]"The Molecular Biology and Anti-genetic Structure of AIDS, ICA, April 15, 1985. [7]At least one lawsuit is in progress against an insurance company denying coverage of an AIDS-related hospitalization claiming that HTLV-III positive anti-body status, as discovered retrospectively for stored sera, constituted a pre-existing condition. The U.S. Army will use positive test results to deny admission to recruits, the *Boston Globe*, 31 August 1985.

## CHAPTER 4

[1]J. Allen McCutchan, et al., University of California at San Diego, "Implications of HTLV-III Antibody Testing for Gay men," at ICA.

[2]NGTF acting director Jeff Levi read the directive at PRM&RC.

[3]Rand L. Stoneburner, New York City Department of Public Health, "Increasing Tuberculosis Incidence and Its Relationship to AIDS in New York City, " at ICA.

[4]Mark E. Whiteside, Institute of Tropical Medicine, Miami, "Outbreak of No-Identifiable-Risk AIDS in Belle Glade, Florida," at ICA.

[5]Jean-Baptiste Brunet, World Health Organization Collaborating Center for AIDS, Paris, reviewed these data including figures cited below in, "The International Occurrence of AIDS," at ICA.

[6]Kenneth Castro, et al., CDC; University of Miami; Downstate Medical Center, Brooklyn, NY in "Risk Factors for AIDS Among Haitians in the U.S.," at ICA. Also, Jean W. Pape, et al., Cheskio, Port-au-Prince, Haiti and Cornell Medical School, New York City in "AIDS in Haiti," at ICA.

[7]R. Ellen Koenig, et al., University Iberoamericano, Santo Domingo, Dominican Republic and University of California at San Diego in "Detection of Antibodies to AIDS-Associated Retrovirus in the Dominican Republic," at ICA.

[8]Jonathan M. Mann, et al., CDC-Atlanta; Mamo Yemo Hospital and Ministry of Health, Kinshasa, Zaire in "Household Transmission of AIDS in Zaire," at ICA.

[9]Nathan Clumeck, et al., St Pierre Hospital, Free University of Brussels, Belgium; University Center of Public Health, Butane, Rwanda in

"Sero-Epidemiological Studies of HTLV-III Antibody Prevalence among Selected Groups of Heterosexual Africans," at ICA.

[10]Martha F. Rogers, et al., CDC-Atlanta; New York City Department of Public Health in "Surveillance for AIDS in Children," at ICA. Also, "Update: AIDS-U.S.," *MMWR*, 30 November 1984, p. 661.

[11]James M. Oleska, et al., UMD-New Jersey Medical School; Children's Hospital of New Jersey; St. Michael's Medical Center, Newark, NJ; St. Joseph's Medical Center, Paterson, N.J.,, "Epidemiological Features of Pediatric AIDS in New Jersey," at ICA.

[12]Gwendolyn B. Scott, et al., University of Miami, Florida, "Mothers and Infants with AIDS: Outcomes of Subsequent Pregnancies," at ICA.

[13]Olesky, *op. cit.*

[14]The most heated part of the controversy arose at an afternoon session on education arranged by the lesbian and gay activists and researchers, in coorperation with other concerned health officials.

[15]See *Mother Jones*, November 1984.

[16]Brunett, op. cit.

[17]Hirsch, op. cit.

## CHAPTER 5

[1]See Michel Foucault, *Birth of the Clinic* (New York: Vintage, 1985), and Ivan Illich, *The Medical Nemesis*, (London: Calder and Boyars, 1975).

[2]William H. McNeill in *Plagues and People* (Garden City: Anchor, 1976), traces the cycles of various epidemics througout Western history.

[3]Astor, op cit., pp. 191-193.

[4]Astor recounts numerous such episodes in recent years. Much of popular medical journalism deals with these "mystery" diseases.

[5]McNeil, op. cit., p. 236.

[6]Foucault, *Birth*, pp. 88-105.

[7]See Susan Sontag, *Illness as Metaphor* (New York: Vintage, 1979).

[8]Barbara Ehrenreich and Deirdre English, *Complaints and Disorders: The Sexual Politics of Sickness* (New York: Feminist Press), p. 39.

[9]Foucault, *Birth*, pp. 107-123.

[10]Alan Sheridan, *Michel Foucault: The Will to Truth* (London and New York: Tavistock, 1982), p. 53, discussing Foucault's *Madness and Civilization*.

[11]Paul Starr's *The Social Transformation of American Medicine* (New York: Basic Books, 1982) details the economic shifts in U.S. medical practice.

[12]See Ehrenreich and English, op. cit. Also Charles E. Rosenberg, *The Cholera Years,* which compares U.S. social attitudes toward cholera in three successive nineteenth-century epidemics.

[13]Starr, op. cit., pp. 47-51.

[14]See DuBois and Gordon, "Seeking Pleasure on the Battlefield," in Carol Vance, ed. *Pleasure and Danger: Exploring Female Sexuality* (Boston and London: Routledge and Kegan Paul, 1984).

[15]Alan Brandt, *No Magic Bullets* (Oxford: Oxford University Press, 1985), pp. 22-23.

[16]See Jeffrey Weeks, *Sex, Politics, and Society: The Regulation of Sexuality Since 1800* (London and New York: Longman, 1981).

[17]The recent work of Weinberg, et al., attempts to show hormonal differences between male homosexuals, male heterosexuals, and female heterosexuals. In addition, a Department of Justice funded research project is attempting to establish hormonal differences in males "susceptible" to pornography.

[18]James Stakely's research on social attitudes and policy toward homosexuality in Nazi Germany has revealed graphs portraying the "spread of homosexuality from the believed tiny minority of "true" homosexuals to "innocent" others. See also, Stakely, *The Homosexual Emancipation Movement in Germany* (New York: Arno Press, 1975).

[19]Both Illich in *Gender* and Foucault in *History of Sexuality* discuss this paradigmatic relationship.

[20]Starr, op. cit., pp. 37-40.

[21]Ibid., pp. 32-34.

[22]Ibid., pp. 116-123.

[23]Barbara Ehrenreich and John Ehrenreich, *The American Health Empire* (New York: Vintage, 1971), pp. 124-132.

[24]Starr, op. cit., pp. 381-388.

[25]Ehrenreich and Ehrenreich, op. cit. p. 107.

[26]Starr, op. cit., pp.127-134.

[27]"Uses of Approved Drugs Unlabelled Uses," *Food and Drug Administration Bulletin,* Volume 12, No. 1, April 1982.

[28]According to letters between the John Hopkins Medical School Institutional Review Board and Depo-Provera researchers.

[29]The *Boston Globe,* 26 January 1983.

[30]*Journal of American Medicine,* 23/30 December 1983.

# CHAPTER 6

[1]Starr, op.cit., p. 389.

²Ibid., p. 410.

³"AIDS: A New Threat to Cops," *The National Centurian*, October 1983. Also, *Corrections Digest*, 27 July 1983, p. 4.

⁴Frances J. Flaherty, "A Legal Emergency Brewing Over AIDS," *National Law Journal*, 9 July 1984, p. 44.

⁵*National Gay STD Service Newsletter*, fall 1984

⁶Lambda, pp. 6-10.

⁷Flaherty, op. cit., p. 44.

⁸Jessica Mitford, *Kind and Unusual Punishment* (New York: Vintage, 1974). Also, Ehrenreich and Ehrenreich, op. cit.

⁹James Jones, *Bad Blood* (New York: Free Press, 1981), pp. 179-190. See also Mitford, op. cit., pp. 163-167.

¹⁰See Jones, op. cit.

¹¹The Belmont Report, 18 April 1979, provides the ethical guidelines for researches. It was developed as mandated by the National Research Act (Publ. 93-348), 12 July 1974, the first law governing research in the U.S. Only in February of 1966 had the Public Health Service even drafted guidelines for the ethical conduct of research. See Jones, op. cit., pp. 189-190.

¹²"A Review of Human Subject Research," *IRB*, November/December 1984, 6.6.

¹³See Jones and Brandt, op. cit.

¹⁴*IRB*, p. 1.

¹⁵See Illich, *Medical Nemesis*. See also a critique of Illich in Leslie Doyal, *The Political Economy of Health* (Boston: South End Press, 1979), pp. 17-21.

¹⁶There was a lengthy discussion of this position at PRIM&R especially by Matilda Krim, a board member of the New York City-based AIDS Medical Foundation, and Alan Novick, professor of medical ethics at Yale University.

¹⁷*Committee on Government operations*, Federal Response to AIDS, p. 207.

¹⁸Lambda, pp. 5-15.

## CHAPTER 7

¹See Harvey Wasserman, *American Born and Re-Born* (New York: Collier, 1983) on the ascendancy of religion and conservatism. See also Sidney Ahlstrom, *A Religious History of the American People* (New Haven and London: Yale University Press, 1972).

²See Edwin Diamond, *Sign Off* (Cambridge: MIT Press, 1982), pp. 29-41, on media technology and the religious right.

[3]H. Richard Neibuhr, *Christ and Culture* (New York: McMillan, 1937), outlines this paradigm for the religious community.

[4]After the 1984 lesbian and gay pride marches, Jerry Falwell sent another of many direct mail packages containing photos of drag queens and men kissing supposedly taken by his son who travelled in cognito in the crowd. The photos are inside a second envelope with the warning, "FOR ADULTS ONLY! Explicit Photographs Enclosed. Please do not let these photos fall into the hands of innocent, impressionable children." Letter is dated 9 August 1984.

[5]American Family Association, 214 Massachusetts Avenue, N.E., Suite 500, Washington D.C. 20002. Letter undated, circa winter 1983.

[6]Christian Family Renewal, P.O. Box 488, Stafford, VA 22554. Letter undated, circa February 1984.

[7]*Southern Medical Journal*, February 1984, pp. 149-150.

[8]D'Emilio, op. cit., p. 19.

[9]Ibid., p. 121.

[10]Christian Anti-Communist Crusade newsletter, 15 January 1984, p. 5.

[11]D'Emilio, op. cit., p. 216.

[12]Alan Crawford, *Thunder on the Right* (New York: Pantheon, 1980), p. 295.

[13]George Gilder, *Wealth and Poverty* (New York: Bantam, 1981), pp.81-82.

[14]Wasserman, op. cit., pp. 232-233.

[15]See *Radical America*, double issue on Rainbow Coalition politics, Volume 17, No. 6/Volume 18, No. 1.

[16]Alert Citizens of Texas, "Homosexuality: The Shattered Image," undated pamphlet, early 1984.

[17]Dr. Ronald Godwin, "AIDS: A Moral and Political Time Bomb," *Moral Majority Report*, July 1982, pp. 2 and 8.

[18]"Be Whole" letter signed by Russell McCraw, May 1984, PO Box 11705, Montgomery Alabama, 36111.

[19]"Prayer Focus," Intercessors for America newsletter, November 1983, PO Box 1289, Elyria, Ohio 44036.

[20]Tearcatchers is a "ministry devoted to training sympathetic sufferers." Its executive director Harold Ivan Smith, author of the AIDS Special Report, specializes in writing for and about living as a single adult (christian). They are non-fundamentalist evangelicals, and identify themselves more closely with christian centrists resisting the hate mongering of ultra-fundamentalists. PO Box 24688, Kansas City, MO 64131. Undated, circa spring 1984.

[21]*Southern Medical Journal*, pp. 149-150.

[22]Cal Thomas, then vice president of the Moral Majority, on their radio show aired 5 February 1982.

[23]Cited, without date, in *Tearcatchers Special Report.*

[24]Gilder, op. cit., p. 90.

[25]Model Sexuality Bill, developed by the Institute for the Scientific Investigation of Sexuality (ISIS), chaired by Dr. Paul Cameron, Lincoln, Nebraska. His "research" is based on door-to-door questionaires. Questions include sexual practices; STD history; drug, alcohol, and tobacco use; cheating on taxes; and "when you knew you had a disease, did you ever have sex with someone to deliberately infect them?" ISIS newsletter, Volume 1, Nos. 1, 2, 3, May 1983-January 1984.

[26]*GAY-AIDS-ERA*, prepared by Eagle Forum. Undated pamphlet, circa winter 1983.

[27]Letter from Jerry Falwell, dated April 1984.

[28]Crawford, op. cit., p.269.

## CHAPTER 8

[1]Carol Vance, ed., op. cit.

[2]"Epilogue." [3]See Robin Ruth Linden, ed., *Against Sado masochism* (Berkeley: Frog In The Well Press, 1982).

[4]Claude Levi-Strauss, *The Raw and the Cooked* (New York: Harper & Row, 1969), and *The Savage Mind* (Chicago: Chicago University Press, 1973).

[5]Gayle Rubin, "Thinking Sex: Notes for a Radical Theory of the Politics of Sexuality," in Carol Vance ed., *Pleasure and Danger.* See also Eve Sedgwick, *Between Men: English Literature and Male Homosocial Desire* (New York: Columbia University Press, 1985).

[6]Consciousness-raising is used widely in Marxist social change movements, but has a specific meaning and context in U.S. movements that differs from European and Central American applications. For the pragmatist roots of this concept, see John E. Smith, *Themes in American Philosophy* (New York: Harper & Row, 1970).

[7]Sheridan, op. cit., p. 180.

[8]*The Advocate*, 7 August 1984, p. 58.

## CHAPTER 9

[1]See K.J. Dorer, *Greek Homosexuality* (New York: Random House, 1980).

[2]See Arthur Evans, *Witchcraft and the Gay Counter-culture* (Boston: Fag

Rag Books, 1978). The Boston Lesbian and Gay History Slideshow documents other cases in Puritan New England.

[3]Stakely elaborates this thesis in his slideshow.

[4]See Lilian Faderman, *Surpassing the Love of Men* (New York: William Morrow & Company, 1981).

[5]The notion of homosexual *acts* versus homosexual *people* has become a cliche of social construction theorists. Jeffrey Weeks is probably due credit for popularizing this idea among British U.S. lesbian/gay scholars.

[6]See Weeks and D'Emilio. Also Alan Berube, "Marching to a Different Drummer," Snitow, et al., eds., *Powers of Desire: The Politics of Sexuality* (New York: Monthly Review Press, 1983).

[7]See Angela Carter, *Sadean Women and the Ideology of Pornography* (New York: Pantheon, 1978).

[8]See Bronski, Weeks, D'Emilio, Boswell.

[9]See Faderman.

[10]There was much discussion of the oppressive nature of butch/fem lesbian relationships in the early years of the women's movement. Recent work, especially by urban working-class and latina lesbians, suggests that butch/fem relationships, although apparently modelling the heterosexual couple, actually contain different meanings. Joan Nestle has written extensively on the subject of butch/fem relationships as positive adaptations to the restrictions placed on urban lesbians, as well as arguing that roles may have been more fluid and not heterosexist as earlier suggested. See Marotta for a historical overview of lesbian feminist views early in the lesbian/gay movement. See Cheri Moraga and Amber Hollibaugh, "What We're Rolling Around in Bed With," in *Powers of Desire.*

[11]See D'Emilio, Weeks, Stakely.

[12]Charles Nelson's controversial novel, *The Boy Who Picked the Bullets Up*, (New York: William Morrow, 1981), recounts gay life among U.S. soldiers during the Viet Nam war. Yokio Mishima's *Forbidden Colors* (New York: Alfred Knopf, 1968) suggests that a well-articulated gay male bar culture, similar to that in the U.S., existed in Japan after World War II.

[13]See Marotta.

[14]Bronski discusses the evolution of the idea of the dandy and its influence on emerging gay male identity. Sedgick also discusses gay male models of behavior in Victorian England, suggesting that images of gay men as masculine versus feminine was a class-linked phenomenon.

[15]See Brandt.

## CHAPTER 10

[1]David G. Ostrow, et al., Northwestern Medical Center, Chicago, "Sexual Behavior Change and Persistence in Homosexual Men," at ICA.

[2]CDC official Donal Francis received a mixed reception for his discussion of separating exposed from non-exposed gay men in the pre-conference seminar on education.

[3]Jill Joseph, et al., University of Michigan, Ann Arbor and Northwestern University Medical Center, Chicago, "Changes in Sexual Behavior of Gay Men: Relationship to Perceived Stress and Psychological Symptomatology," at ICA.

[4]*First Hand, Drummer,* and *Manscape* have all made an effort to include both accurate information and encouragement..

[5]Alan R. Kristal, "Can Legislation to Close Bathhouses Reduce AIDS Incidents? An Epidemological Analysis of Atrributable Risk," at ICA.

[6]Joseph, et al., op.cit.

## CHAPTER 11

[1]Mike Reigle, "The Fens: A Sexual and Political Cruise," *Gay Community News,* 1 October 1983.

[2]Scott Tucker, "Tinkerbell Meets Trotsky," *Gay Community News,* October Book Supplement, 1981. He reviews two unauthorized pamphlets of internal documents on the homosexual question.

[3]See *Powers of Desire* for a range of articles on class and sexuality. See also Weeks for a theoretical overview.

[4]The Alternative Press Index provides a listing for "AIDS" and is the most up-to-date single resource on progressive publications.

# Bibliography

Ahlstrom, Sydney E. *A Religious History of the American People.* New Haven, London: Yale University Press, 1972.

Albert, Michael, and Robin Hahnel. *Marxism and Socialist Theory.* Boston: South End Press, 1981.

Ackerman, Frank. *Reaganomics: Rhetoric vs. Reality.* Boston: South End Press, 1982.

*American Psychologist.* "Psychology in the Public Forum: Series on AIDS." November 1984, Vol. 39, No. 11.

Astor, Gerald. *The Disease Detectives.*New York: Plume, 1983.

Boswell, John. *Christianity, Social Tolerance and Homosexuality.* Chicago: University of Chicago Press, 1980.

Brandt, Alan. *No Magic Bullets.* London: Oxford University Press, 1985.

Bronski, Michael. *Culture Clash: The Making of a Gay Sensibility.* Boston: South End Press, 1984.

Carter, Angela. *The Sadean Woman and the Ideology of Pornography.* New York: Pantheon, 1978.

Committee on Government Operations, U.S. House of Representatives, 98th Congress. *Federal Response to AIDS.* Washington: Government Printing Office, 1983.

Crawford, Alan. *Thunder on the Right.* New York: Pantheon, 1980.

Curtis, Zelda. "'Private' Lives and Communism," *The Left and the Erotic,* ed. Eileen Phillips. London: Lawrence and Wishart, 1983.

D'Emilio, John. *Sexual Politics, Sexual Communities.* Chicago: University of Chicago Press, 1983.

Diamond, Edwin. *Sign Off.* Cambridge: MIT Press, 1982.

Dorer, K.J. *Greek Homosexuality.* New York: Random House, 1980.

175

Douglas, Mary. *Purity and Danger*. London: Routledge and Kegan Paul, 1978.

Doyal, Lesley. *The Political Economy of Health*. Boston: South End Press, 1979.

Ehrenreich, Barbara. *Hearts of Men*. Garden City, N.Y.: Doubleday, 1983.

———and John Ehrenreich. *The American Health Empire: Report of Health/PAC*. New York: Vintage, 1971.

——— and Deirdre English. *Complaints and Disorders: The Sexual Politics of Sickness*. Old Westbury, N.Y.: Feminist Press, 1973.

———, Karin Stallard, and Holly Sklar. *Poverty in the American Dream: Women and Children First*. Boston: South End Press, 1983.

Evans, Arthur. *Witchcraft and the Gay Counter-culture*. Boston: Fag Rag Books, 1978.

Faderman, Lillian. *Surpassing the Love of Men*. New York: William Morrow, 1981.

Foucault, Michel. *The Birth of the Clinic*. New York: Vintage, 1975.

——— *Power/Knowledge*. New York: Pantheon, 1980.

——— *The History of Sexuality, Vol. 1*. New York: Vintage, 1980.

Freud, Sigmund. *Civilization and Its Discontents*. New York: W.W. Norton, 1961.

Gilder, George. *Wealth and Poverty*. New York: Bantam, 1981.

Harris, Marvin. *The Rise of Anthropological Thought*. New York: Thomas Crowell, 1968.

——— *America Now*. New York: Simon and Schuster, 1981.

Hunter, Alan. "In the Wings: New Right Organization and Ideology," *Radical America*, Spring 1981, Vol. 15, Nos. 1 and 2.

Illich, Ivan. *Gender*. New York: Pantheon, 1982.

——— *Medical Nemesis*. London: Calder and Boyars, 1975.

Jezer, Marty. *The Dark Ages: Life in the U.S. 1945—1960*. Boston: South End Press, 1982.

Jones, James H. *Bad Blood*. New York: Free Press, 1981.

Knowler, Louis, and Kenneth Prewitt. *Institutional Racism in America*. Englewood Cliffs, N.J.: Prentice-Hall, 1969.

Kuhn, Thomas. *The Structure of Scientific Revolutions*. Chicago: University of Chicago Press, 1970.

Lambda Legal Defense and Education Fund. *AIDS Legal Guide*. 132 W. 43rd St., New York, NY 10036. 1984.

Loach, Edmund. *Claude Levi-Strauss*. New York: Penguin, 1976.

Levi-Strauss, Claude. *The Savage Mind*. Chicago: University of Chicago Press, 1973.

———— *Totemism*. Boston: Beacon, 1963.

———— *The Raw and the Looked*. New York: Harper and Row, 1969.

Linden, Robin Ruth, ed. *Against Sado-masochism*. Berkeley: Frog in the Well, 1982.

Marcuse, Herbert. *Counter-revolution and Revolt*. Boston: Beacon, 1972.

Marotta, Toby. *The Politics of Homosexuality*. Boston: Houghton Mifflin, 1981.

Mayer, Ken, and Hank Pizer. *The AIDS Fact Book*. 1982.

McNeill, William H. *Plagues and People*. Garden City, N.Y.: Anchor, 1976.

Mishima, Yukio. *Forbidden Colors*. New York: Alfred A. Knopf, 1968.

Mitford, Jessica. *Kind and Usual Punishment: The Prison Business*. New York: Vintage, 1974.

Nelson, Charles. *The Boy Who Picked the Bullets Up*. New York: William Morrow, 1981.

Niebuhr, H. Richard. *Christ and Culture*. New York: McMillan, 1937.

Ollman, Bertell. *Social and Sexual Revolution*. Boston: South End Press, 1979.

Parran, Thomas. *Shadow on the Land*. New York: Reynal and Hitchcock, 1937.

Piaget, Jean. *Psychology and Epistemology*. New York: Viking, 1970.

———— *Structuralism*. New York: Harper and Row, 1968.

Quebedeaux, Richard. *By What Authority*. San Francisco: Harper and Row, 1981.

Rofes, Eric. *I Thought People Like That Killed Themselves*. San Francisco: Grey Fox Press, 1982.

Rosebury, Theodor. *Microbes and Morals*. New York: Viking, 1971.

Rosenburg, Charles E. *The Cholera Years*. Chicago: University of Chicago Press, 1962.

Rubin, Gayle. "The Traffic in Women: Notes on the 'Political Economy' of Sex," *Toward an Anthropology of Women*, ed. Rayna Reiter. New York: Monthly Review Press, 1975.

Ryan, William. *Blaming the Victim*. New York: Vintage, 1971.

Sahlins, Marshall. *The Use and Abuse of Biology*. Ann Arbor: Univeristy of Michigan Press, 1976.

Sedgewick, Eve Rosofsky. *Between Men: English Literature and Male Homosexual Desire*. New York: Columbia University Press, 1985.

Sheridan, Alan. *Michel Foucault: The Will to Truth.* London: Tunistock, 1982.

Siegal, Frederick and Marta. *AIDS: The Medical Mystery.* New York: Grove, 1983.

*Signs.* "French Feminist Theory," Autumn 1981, Vol. 7, No. 1.

Smith, John E. *Themes in American Philosophy.* New York: Harper and Row, 1970.

———— *The Spirit of American Philosophy.* London: Oxford University Press, 1963.

Snitow, Ann, Christine Stansell, and Sharon Thompson, eds. *Powers of Desire: The Politics of Sexuality.* New York: Monthly Review Press, 1983.

Sontag, Susan. *Illness As Metaphor.* New York: Vintage, 1979.

Stakely, James. *The Homosexual Emancipation Movement in Germany.* New York: Arno Press, 1975.

Starr, Paul. *The Social Transformation of American Medicine.* New York: Basic Books, 1982.

Totman, Richard. *Social Causes of Illness.* New York: Pantheon, 1979.

Vance, Carol, ed. *Pleasure and Danger: exploring female sexuality.* London: Routledge and Kegan Paul, 1984.

Wasserman, Harvey. *America Born and Reborn.* New York: Collier, 1983.

Weeks, Jeffrey. *Sex, Politics, and Society: The Regualtion of Sexuality Since 1800.* London: Congman, 1981.

Williams, Raymond. *Culture and Society: 1780—1950.* New York: Columbia University Press, 1983.

# Index